THEROUX THE KEYHOLE

LOUIS THEROUX

PAN BOOKS

First published 2021 by Macmillan

This paperback edition first published 2022 by Pan Books
an imprint of Pan Macmillan
The Smithson, 6 Briset Street, London EC1M 5NR
EU representative: Macmillan Publishers Ireland Ltd, 1st Floor,
The Liffey Trust Centre, 117–126 Sheriff Street Upper,
Dublin 1, D01 YC43
Associated companies throughout the world
www.panmacmillan.com

ISBN 978-1-5098-8045-4

1 3 5 7 9 8 6 4 2

A CIP catalogue record for this book is available from the British Library.

Typeset in Warnock Pro by Jouve (UK), Milton Keynes
Printed and bound by CPI Group (UK) Ltd, Croydon, CR0 4YY

Visit **www.panmacmillan.com** to read more about all our books
and to buy them. You will also find features, author interviews and
news of any author events, and you can sign up for e-newsletters
so that you're always first to hear about our new releases.

For my family

Contents

In times of peace, the warlike man attacks himself.
Friedrich Nietzsche

Never easy, burpees. Never easy.
Joe Wicks

PREFACE TO THE PAPERBACK EDITION

Hello and welcome to the paperback version of *Theroux the Keyhole*! You have in your hands a product much like the hardback, but smaller, bendier and less expensive. It contains all the words that were included in the original publication, but also – *try to remain calm* – some *bonus material*.

Yes, despite the reduced size, it is in fact *more book*.

I write this preface – masked, in Phoenix airport, awaiting a plane – some six months or so after the hardback's publication. I am in the departure lounge, where I have just eaten an unsatisfactory McDonald's (Deluxe Crispy Chicken Sandwich, the chicken tasted weird to me), and I have a moment to reflect on what it was like writing my book and then putting it out into the world.

Theroux the Keyhole started as an attempt to chronicle the first lockdown. Soon after it was announced the world was going on hiatus due to the onset of a global pandemic, I thought someone should make notes on all the weird stuff that was happening. And why shouldn't that someone be me? At school, studying history, I used to read chronicles by anonymous monks in the Middle Ages writing about Viking raids. I also enjoyed the jottings of later figures like John Aubrey, Samuel Pepys and Michel de Montaigne, talking about random intimate details of their life like their sleeping habits and indigestion. Maybe this would be my contribution to the genre of 'random dude writes stuff about his life that might be interesting in 500 years'.

I carried on writing it as the Covid situation got worse, then better, then worse again . . . The book evolved into a portrait of my family life and also a behind-the-scenes record of the work that was preoccupying me: putting together a TV series, some podcast interviews, a special about Joe Exotic, and some other stuff.

At times, while writing it, I wasn't sure whether it was any good. But I banished those thoughts and kept going, piling up entries on a more or less nightly basis, sometimes sober, sometimes under the influence of a few drinks. I tried to record direct speech and sketch small domestic scenes of conflict and humour. As I read back over previous entries, at times it seemed to me I was accumulating an unflinching portrait of naked humanity, of astonishing honesty – a portrait of a writer and his family that in a small way extended the frontier of literature. Other times, it seemed I'd written a load of trivial shit. Perhaps there isn't that much difference? (*Dun-dun-dun!*)

I told myself that we have people backwards, valuing them based on their work, when in fact their true self is the one they keep hidden: the rage-prone and erratic private individual, not the one that wins the Nobel Prize for Physics. This book would be an antidote to that kind of curating of a public persona. It's definitely the case that when I think about books I've enjoyed, it's often the small intimacies I've connected with.

We know Shakespeare was a great playwright, but what was he like when Hamnet was acting up and wouldn't finish his capon, or Judith wanted to stay up late playing with her wooden cup-and-ball? Did he and Anne Hathaway take turns stuffing the goose, and did she have an issue with how much 'sack' he drank during the plague year of 1592? Because that's what I want to know.

(And, yes, I just compared myself to Shakespeare.)

After a year of writing, I had about 140,000 words. With my editor, I cut out about half of the material. I rewrote the entries, trimming and merging them, to make it flow better.

When I published it, I was confident the book would find a receptive audience and maybe be widely reviewed. In fact, it was only reviewed in one place that I'm aware of. I'm pretty sure no one took the view that I had extended the frontier of literature.

In writing the book, it was my aim to be as honest as possible about my shortcomings as a husband and parent. I hold the view that we are, all of us, more mixed up and messy than we let on, but that by being honest about our failings, we can connect with one another and try to be better. I've been pleased to hear from people who've read it that they were surprised at 'how honest' I was.

So here I am, six months on from publication, and nearly two years since I started writing. Flicking through this smaller, bendier edition, I actually think it holds up OK. Parts of it make me cringe to read. It may have done my reputation no favours, sharing all this. But maybe that's the point. Being stupid and being honest about it. That's my hope, anyway. If you think I come across as embarrassing, rage-prone, cringe – choose your adjective – I don't disagree.

Right, that's my flight being called. I better wrap this up. Mainly I want to say thanks for checking out the book. I hope you enjoy it. And also, in general, at McDonald's, it's probably better to go burger, not chicken.

Prologue

Man Bites Pangolin

After fifteen minutes of 'remote learning', Ray, aged six, has already had enough. The video-conferencing app is malfunctioning, and the teacher's voice is doing a weird echo thing reminiscent of an effect they used on dub reggae records in the eighties. *OK, children. KRONG-KRONG-KRONG-krong-krong!! Is everyone muted? DOD-DOD-DOD-dod-dod!!*

'I'm bored,' Ray says. 'What can I doo-oo?'

A few feet away, at the end of the kitchen table, I am wrenched away from the past-deadline TV treatment I am supposed to be writing, shocked by sudden stabs of despair and rage. A tiny still-calm part of my mind reflects on the surprising violence of what I'm feeling and the strangeness that the simple act of supervising schoolwork from home should be quite so crazy-making. It considers the many places I'd rather be: behind bars in the ad-seg wing of a large maximum-security prison; enduring a tongue-lashing from the demented guru of a cult in the Midwest; in Leeds huffing the cigar breath of a famous serial sexual predator.

Anywhere but here.

Eighteen months into the planetary pandemic, our three children have been sent home *again* because someone – a teacher, a fellow pupil – has tested positive. Nancy, my wife, is run ragged, verging on nervous collapse, on the rack of unrealistic work commitments, her own health not 100 per cent following a dalliance with the virus. Nieces, nephews, and two brothers-in-law are all ill, laid low by the Delta variant. And a few days ago word came that videos are travelling around TikTok, the sinister social media platform and data-harvesting tool, showing children how to hack their Covid tests with lemon juice so they can produce false positives and get themselves out of school. It turns out this latest bout of mayhem may all be down to some work-shy kids and a bottle of Jif Squeezy.

Like America, bombed at Pearl Harbor, the family Theroux finds itself dragged into a conflict it did not want, fighting on several fronts – against the virus, against inconsistent and confusing measures intended to subdue the virus, against disinformation, against screen addiction, against an inability to agree on what we would all like to watch on TV.

A year and a half of madness has left its marks, even in the gilded world of a documentary presenter – the Dame Vera Lynn of Lockdown Podcasting™. Drinking too much, prone to embarrassing rages, losses of control and absent-mindedness, as well as feelings of inadequacy that may be the inevitable lot of a father trying to do his best, always on the verge of being 'cringe'. Did I mention drinking too much?

I look back at the period of house arrest we've been forced into – granted, with a few transatlantic work trips thrown in – like a general surveying the ruined landscape of the territory he's conquered, pockmarked with the figurative scars of children going mental, squabbling and fighting, spending weeks on end without seeing friends, a beautiful and supportive wife grief-stricken at her lack of contact with the outside world, and the paterfamilias – that being me – who was confused and irresolute, and at times even weirdly appreciative of some aspects of the crisis, perhaps feeling that he needed to make his peace and get along with his new planetary roommate, the virus, since it wasn't showing signs of leaving, or maybe he was just too lacking in self-knowledge to know exactly *what* he was feeling half the time?

We may be near the end of this thing. We may not be. I'll say this for my friend Covid-19: it is full of surprises, and the good news is we have plenty of Greek letters on hand for its next David Bowie-like act of shape-shifting. Early in the whole adventure, in mid-March 2020, realizing we were entering an era of memorable weirdness, I began keeping a diary, which I continued for exactly a year. My decision to look back now may prove premature and hopelessly irrelevant, especially if a Sigma variant arrives that is more contagious and more debilitating, and is wearing plat-form heels with a red lightning bolt painted across its face. But if twenty-five years spent documenting the fringes of life and the most extreme forms of existential angst have taught me anything, it's that often in the darkest times we find the most meaningful connection. So here I am, letting my readers in on a story that doesn't unfold in any of my usual journalistic feeding grounds of a porn set or a militia compound or a maximum-security psychiatric unit, but instead on a frontier much closer to home, one that has been the site of more stress and more fear – for me, at least – than any other I've reported from, which is to say, my house, during a pandemic.

• • •

On the morning of New Years's Eve 2019, I was pottering around in my kitchen in north-west London listening to the radio when a news item came on about a disease in Wuhan, China, linked to some kind of meat market called a 'wet market', a phrase I'd never heard before that struck me as faintly grotesque. For a moment, I wondered why we were being told that someone 10,000 miles away had caught a virus, and why was it more important than all the other people who must be ill in China, in Darfur, or indeed on Willesden High Road. But presumably the editors of BBC Radio 4's *Today* programme knew their business – it was news for a reason – and my mind drifted, and I got on with other things.

It had been a busy holiday. We had taken over Christmas hosting duties from Nancy's mum at late notice, because of a family illness. Nancy, on top of all organizing and coordinating of guests, was also in charge of the main meal. My job was the potatoes, which were, if I say so myself, a triumph – par-boiled and shaken roughly in the pan to fluff them up, drizzled in olive oil, and then roasted into crispy golden perfection. I had ferried bottles of wine around for the guests – 'Can I freshen you up?' – while swatting at my son Jack, who despite being twelve years old was attempting to cadge some for himself, ever curious to try anything with the cachet of the forbidden. 'Just a little sip, Dad, go on.' After lunch with crackers and paper hats and the aforementioned magical potatoes, we'd had a kickabout in the garden, then slumped in the front room and watched whatever was on TV. There was, naturally, a Christmas tree that our youngest son Ray had helped to decorate. We had put stockings out the night before, evoking the Yuletide magic in the appropriate fashion for a five-year-old. 'Don't forget carrots for the reindeer and some brandy for Santa . . .' All three boys had put up stockings, even Arthur, who was fourteen and had made emphatic references to the mysterious workings of Saint Nick and his ability to defy physics and descend chimneys many times narrower than his girth, partly out of respect for Ray, but also mindful of not wanting his own Christmas privileges called into question.

Nancy and I had had our traditional argument over why I hadn't been more involved in getting gifts for the kids – me thinking, though trying hard not to say, that if I could have taken some of their presents back to the shop, to decrease the number of their gifts, I would have been happy to. A thought partly born out of stinginess, but mainly out of a puritanical disapproval of excess and a sadness that ensued whenever I saw new possessions freed from their gift wrap only to grow old in a matter of hours, lose their magic, and become more clutter.

'When I was growing up we had presents in the leg of a pair of tights and none of them were wrapped, and we were fine with it,' I'd said.

'OK, but I didn't.'

'They're supposed to be little tokens, not actual gifts. Satsumas and nuts and pencil sharpeners. Stuff like that.'

'I'm sure they'd love to come down on Christmas morning and find a stocking full of nuts,' Nancy had said. 'Stop being a grinch, Louis.'

In the months leading up to Christmas I'd been more than usually preoccupied with work. Nancy and I had recently taken the leap of launching a new company, which – following months of dithering about possible names – we'd called Mindhouse. Twenty-five years of toiling within the BBC had ended; I was now making programmes independently. The creation of Mindhouse had been a dream long in gestation, in equal measure exciting and stressful. The creative opportunities – the chance to make series I wasn't in, single documentaries, shows featuring other presenters – went hand in hand with more financial risk. It had been Nancy's idea to take the leap. We'd met at the BBC, where she had made documentaries in the history department. She'd taken time out of her career to have our children and was now ready to get back into full-time programme-making. Our starting a company was, among other things, an opportunity for us to work together. Though, if I was completely honest, there was a part of it that terrified me: the idea of putting strain on our relationship, professional as well as personal, and creating a situation in which we would have no escape from one another, no respite, when the going got tough either at home or at work.

In November 2019, we'd taken up occupancy of some offices in Shepherd's Bush and begun work on a series of ideas, including a new possible three-parter which I would present, on the theme of 'radicalization'. For years I'd had an interest in the far right in America, and lately I'd been following a new online underground of young gamers and trolls who lurked in a bulletin board called 4chan, sharing racist memes and tasteless jokes about child suicides. I'd also been tracking the homegrown jihadis stuck in limbo in northern Iraq and Syria, people who'd left the UK to take part in the dream of the ISIS caliphate, and were now stateless and to varying degrees remorseful of having joined a medieval death cult. Both these stories struck me as saying something about the strange world we now lived in, in which extremist content could be piped into bedrooms anywhere in the world – where the lines of irony and sincerity, role play and real life were blurred – with potentially disastrous consequences for those on the receiving end.

Alongside them was a third idea about SoundCloud rap in Florida, a musical subgenre often involving depressive lyrics, prescription drugs, and facial tattoos. I was aware the rap story sat oddly alongside the jihadis and the far right, and didn't really fit the brief of 'radicalization', though it was also true that some of the more outrageous behaviour associated with the scene was turbocharged by the possibilities of social media and live streaming: rappers getting inked with garish images and provocative words on their foreheads and cheeks to drive clicks on Instagram and consuming epic quantities of drugs on their feeds knowing it would engage fans.

After several years of making programmes in a minor key – about eating disorders, psychosis, the terminally ill – I hoped the radicalization series would be a return to a weirder, more brightly hued story, with arguments and danger. I'd treated these subjects in the past, in programmes I'd made in my twenties and thirties, but it seemed to me the world had moved on, and I'd moved on, and we were now in a futuristic landscape I could never have imagined when I was a young man. A world where extremism no longer existed merely on the fringes of the culture or in the darkest part of our most poisonous impulses, but instead freely travelled social-media platforms. In the US, we had a president who had tweeted his way into the White House, sending his messages directly to the smartphones of tens of millions of Americans. The utopian promise of an open internet with free access to information had evolved into something more complicated: exciting, transgressive, misinformed, narcissistic, occasionally hateful. Political and social division was at an all-time high, and the paradoxical lesson one was tempted to draw was that instead of pulling us together, our era of technological interconnectedness had created a golden age of tribalism and barbarity.

• • •

For the last few days of the Christmas break we were in Bath with some American friends. We stayed in an Airbnb in the old part of town, having ridden up on the train. We took walks around the city, visited the Jane Austen museum and the famous baths, and their museum, where we all wandered wordlessly, each with our Acoustiguide pressed to one ear: *number 47 . . . you are standing in the frigidarium, the best preserved of the ancient aqua features . . .* The museum had press-ganged the American author Bill Bryson into recording off-the-cuff thoughts which you could hear if you pushed certain buttons. *The carving in the keystone of the bearded old man is wonderful. He reminds me somehow of a farmer . . . I like his twinkling eyes.*

On our last day we trekked up the tower of Bath Abbey, where the bell rang twelve times and I made a joke about how pleasurable it was being close to so many enormous dongs.

Then came a series of live shows I was doing down under – on 6 January I left the family for two weeks, landing in Auckland, and from there visiting Perth, Adelaide and Sydney. All this time, in the background, was the apocalyptic drumbeat – not of the coronavirus, which was barely mentioned, but of rampant forest fires caused by climate change, leading to the deaths of millions of animals. The final date of the tour, in Melbourne, was in a convention centre. There were two performances, with around 4,000 people in the audience for each. I'd done a live tour once before and I had the same sensation of stepping into someone else's life, a more successful doppelganger, and of feeling slightly fraudulent, serving myself up to audiences who were so appreciative that the 'me' they met surely had to be a disappointment. I reminded myself of a dubious televangelist or self-help guru, and part of me questioned the whole set-up, but the greater part of me loved it, while also wondering whether I might be in danger of tipping into full-blown egomania. Or did the fact that I was concerned about it mean I was managing to keep the egomania in check?

The weeks after were a return to civilian life in the darkness of London in winter, with the daily cycles to and from work – I'd listen to podcasts about the far right and the Internet and the need to deplatform certain speakers who were promoting hate or equally persuasive arguments for safeguarding freedom of speech from censorious busybodies terrified of being exposed to an opinion they disagreed with. There were meetings with other presenters I admired who I hoped we might work with and brainstorming sessions on ideas for box sets and true-crime stories.

Recce trips went ahead – a director and producer flew out to America to meet with potential interviewees for my radicalization series. There was a gentle rising gradient of concern about what was happening in Wuhan. It was reported that the likeliest origin of the virus was someone there eating a weird animal, probably a bat, and on right-wing Twitter gruesome photos circulated of what appeared to be a Chinese woman eating bat soup, with a little bat carcass perched on the edge of her bowl. Later the photos were revealed to be three years old and taken thousands of miles away on the Pacific island of Palau. Reports from Italy and Iran suggested the virus was spreading, but the numbers still sounded small and the situation never seemed likely to disturb us or make us change our plans. My preoccupations were more prosaic ones: Would the programmes turn out OK? Would our new company win other commissions? Was I drinking too much? Was this my life?

March 2020

LOCKDOWN

Tuesday 17 March

The first visible sign of panic: the supermarkets. No pasta, no tinned tomatoes, no tinned beans. Yesterday at the Queen's Park Co-op the cashier said: 'People come in yesterday, the day before, clear them out.' Today at pick-up at the primary school, another parent, a dad who works in catering, was saying he'd laid in some extra supplies from a cash and carry in Cricklewood called Bestway: 5 kg bags of penne pasta that he was selling at cost. 'They have big bags of rice too,' his wife said. 'Nancy says you're interested.' Another mum mentioned rumours that wine and spirits were running out.

'Grey Goose converted their facility to produce rubbing alcohol,' Catering Dad said.

'There's no vodka anywhere, apparently,' the mum said. 'People are buying it to use as a disinfectant.'

'Yeh,' Catering Dad said. 'Which doesn't work, by the way. The alcohol content's not high enough.'

I bought a 5 kg bag of pasta, out of the back of his van, in front of the school, and then five packets of corn for popping. *Ray will like these*, I thought. And then, with a little squirt of excitement: *This feels a little like maybe what they did during rationing.*

It all started escalating last week. On Monday 9 March, the Italian government imposed a nationwide lockdown. No sports events, travel allowed only for family emergencies. There were photos in the paper of deserted tourist attractions. More than 400 deaths in Italy alone.* Still, somehow, I remained in denial about what was going on. *It won't affect me. Life will go on.* I didn't think about where it

* Daily case and death figures are as reported at the time and from my own notes.

might lead, just enjoyed the spectacle of something different, that little jolt of excitement I used to get at primary school when the fire alarm went off, a departure from the routine, as I gawped at the photos online and reflected on the strangeness of something that still seemed far away.

On Saturday night, Nancy had gone for a long-planned girls' weekend in the West Country. I was left holding the fort. Three kids, on my own. A tiny payback for all the many months I've spent travelling for work while she's been at home. It doesn't often happen, as Nancy likes to point out. My brother Marcel had invited me and the kids over for the night at his house in Tooting, which naturally I seized on as a chance to take some pressure off.

On the drive south, Arthur and Jack were fighting in the back of the car, while Ray threw a fit because the iPad didn't have 3G and couldn't stream YouTube. 'Can one of you please connect the iPad to your personal hotspot? *Guys!*' Jack was already annoyed because I wanted to catch up on the news and had refused to put Capital XTRA on.

'I can't share my data, I don't have any left,' he said. 'Why don't you do it, Ticky?' For obscure reasons, this was something he'd begun calling Arthur.

'Jack, you're so selfish.'

'Stop waffling, Arthur, it's not that deep.'

Nancy called in on the hands-free and asked how it was going.

'We're heading south. Marce invited me over.'

'Oh, I see. Already running for help,' she teased.

'Well, he invited us over. Was I supposed to refuse, just to prove a point?'

On the radio, all the news was Covid-related. Flights were being restricted, new guidelines coming out. We should be washing our hands frequently, ideally for twenty seconds, they said, the same time it took to sing 'Happy Birthday' twice. Avoid touching your face or shaking hands. Numbers were going up in Iran. There was a gathering storm, an ominous mood music, but no clear sense of where it was all going.

At Marcel's house, we sat in the kitchen. I drank a couple of gin and tonics and we caught up, striking up new phrases with an air of novelty.

'I'm supposed to be flying on Monday but it's not clear we'll be able to go.'

I sensed I didn't have his full attention. He looked at me and said, 'Lot of face touching going on.'

'Don't worry, I've washed my hands.'

'How long for?'

I'd brought a melanzane alla parmigiana I'd made. Friends arrived, a newspaper editor and a TV presenter, and we made conversation about the news – projects they'd been working on, the divisiveness running through different cultural debates, an argument within feminism about trans activism that was causing ructions at the editor's workplace, old-guard feminists wanting to preserve a distinction between women and trans women – the debate was highly charged, much of it taking place on social media. I mentioned my plans for new shows – the 'radicalization' series, a big ambitious shoot, finally getting under way after months of planning – but that it was all up in the air now. Updates kept coming in and the situation seemed ever more doubtful, with more restrictions being announced for visitors to the US.

Adding urgency was the knowledge that Mindhouse, as a company, was financially exposed. We'd put money into development. There were also schedule issues. One of the key figures in the far-right film, a baby-faced twenty-something named Nicholas J. Fuentes who was emerging as the new leader of white nationalism in America, was planning an event, a gathering of radicals and self-described dissidents. If we postponed shooting we'd miss it.

A text came in from Nancy saying we needed to have a conference call – me and her, and our two company partners, Arron and Sophie. I phoned in from the staircase of the house, tuning out the sounds of people chatting and doors opening and closing. Arron was fresh from a conversation with our BBC commissioner.

'She thinks it's a bad idea,' he said. 'If we go and one of you gets ill or you can't get back, they're saying it's on us, basically. But if we follow their suggestion to postpone, they'll help us with costs and stuff like that.'

'I don't want to be a dick about it,' I said. 'But I'd like to file a dissenting opinion.'

The gin and tonics were making their presence felt and I was conscious of not being totally with it. I wondered if this was one of those occasions when I was supposed to show leadership, which isn't my strong suit at the best of times. The truth was, I had a strong urge to fly. The idea that we'd be one of the last teams into the US was, to my booze-clouded mind, a reason to go. We could steal a march on the competition, scooping up material while they were all locked out, then come back with the satisfying feeling of being ahead of the game. When I was younger, I used to get the same sensation going into work on a Sunday when the office was empty or during the World Cup.

'I can't see why, if we can get out there and film, we wouldn't do that?'

'Getting out there isn't the issue,' Arron said. 'It's getting back. You could be stuck in a hotel in America for weeks, unable to film and unable to come back.'

'Right, got you,' I said. 'So it's a risk.'

When it was his bedtime, I went up with Ray and read a story, and lay with him until he was asleep. Then came back down to talk some more, turning in with the older children, and the following morning drove back to north-west London. When Nancy arrived back, all three children were, miraculously, still alive, uninjured, with their full complement of teeth, though I tried not to make too big a thing out of it, being resigned by now to the idea that the days I'd been away for work are a debt I will never be able to pay off. The following morning, on Monday, I went into work as usual. By now it was clear the decision to travel or not to travel had been taken away from us; there would be no filming trip to America anytime soon, and maybe the only surprising part was that it was taking me so long to wrap my head around the fact that everything was changing.

Today, after dropping off Ray, I'd headed into the office. Most of our staff are already working from home, as advised by the government. I wandered up and down the corridors, opening doors using my shirt sleeves. In an open-plan area in the centre of the building is a cafe called Coterie. Under a glass vitrine, there were displays of croissants and muffins with rhubarb, and luxury cookies, and it made me sad to think that they might all have to be thrown away. The manager, a Middle Eastern man in middle age, circled above them with an air of tragedy.

Wednesday 18 March

First day working from home.

The good part about being forced to work at home is that the anxiety and the urge to engage in displacement activity mean you get little jobs done. I spent an hour in the morning organizing the wires behind the TV and the set-top box and the DVD player and the PlayStation in the front room, making them look less like a mass of knots and tangles. I used rubber bands to tie them up, then found a smart little box to put miscellaneous wires and accessories into.

For work, we are trying to think of ideas that don't involve travel or meeting people, which feels – for someone whose brand involves travelling and meeting people – a rather restrictive brief.

EastEnders has been suspended, and *Graham Norton*. On social media, there are videos of shirtless English lager louts in southern Spain defying official guidance and refusing to leave the streets, pushing trolleys full of beer and chanting 'We've all got the virus'. Meanwhile, somewhere in East Asia, parents confined indoors have created small obstacle courses for their children: four-year-olds doing calisthenics in tiny apartments. Everywhere, photos of empty shelves in supermarkets and videos of squabbles over toilet paper. Seeing an opening, I tweeted, 'I have some toilet paper if anyone needs any. It is used but only on one side', for a handy 19,000 likes. Online video content is our version of the wartime Victrola radio set. Someone has mocked up a Where's Wally? coronavirus edition, in which you have to spot the woolly hatted beanpole man. He is the only person on an empty street.

Many on the Twitterverse are showing their Blitz spirit, rallying around in the common cause of pouring loathing on a video of Hollywood actors singing a very out of tune version of 'Imagine'. It was started by Gal Gadot, as a way of lifting the spirits of the public, which it did, but perhaps not in the way she intended.

In the afternoon, a friend of Jack's came over. He mentioned that he has various allergies. Eggs, dairy, nuts. But not peanuts. 'I think it's because they're not nuts,' he said. 'They're a *legoon*.'

As we ate supper, we talked about nuts in general. 'I like walnuts,' I said.

Jack said, 'Dad, they are literally the most cringe nuts you can like.'

'I also like almonds.'

'Almonds are like BTEC walnuts,' Jack said.

Nancy said there are pictures on the Internet of the water in Venice running clear for the first time in decades, with fish frolicking and gambolling in the shadow of the Bridge of Sighs. So there's that.

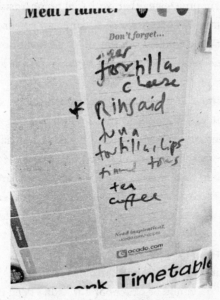

During the rinse aid crisis.

Thursday 19 March

For the first time in recent memory, Ray was pleased to be going to school. This was because 'red class' and 'blue class' have been merged due to low attendance. We have been in a routine where I carry him from the car to the classroom and then he has to be prised off me like a limpet while I run out the door. But today he got down of his own accord and wandered in and then started colouring with his friends. He asked me to bring him a 'kit-e-kat' at pick-up. Meaning Kit-Kat. 'OK,' I said. 'If you promise to be good.' I couldn't bear to correct his pronunciation. Nancy, who was also there, widened her eyes and mouthed: *No more chocolate at pick-up.*

Afterwards I filled up the car at the local garage, then went to the Co-op for milk. With everything going on, it seems less urgent to get into work on time, given that work is at home. Inside the Co-op, no pasta or tinned veg but plenty of wine and spirits. A man in a mask speaking in a muffled voice said to another shopper, 'I don't know if it's true but they were saying a million people lost their jobs yesterday.'

'I know, I know. Strange times,' the woman said.

Yesterday it was announced that on-site learning for Jack and Arthur will end after today. Ray will have his last day tomorrow. Also, today, something about all exams being cancelled. Euro 2020 has been pushed back a year. The Tokyo Olympics are still on for now. The older boys were in uproar because we mentioned that homeschool did *not* mean them being on phones and PlayStation all day every day.

'*What?* But we're not at school!' Jack said.

'Well, you are at school, but you're doing it at home. Got it? You're at home, but you would be at school if it hadn't been cancelled.'

'You're literally not making any sense.'

Only last week this all seemed as though it might be over in a few weeks. Earlier this week, I'd mentally revised that to May or June. Now there are whispers, unconfirmed, that children may be out of school until September. Yet reports from China last night said that there were no new cases of Covid yesterday for the first time.

We were supposed to announce our new production company signing a deal with BBC Studios but now that seems badly timed. With people being laid off and, you know, dying.

My brother called up to chat. Earlier in the week he'd sent me a parody song of his devising, 'My Corona', based on 'My Sharona' by The Knack, and to lift our spirits we brainstormed other ideas for comical songs themed around the pandemic.

'I was thinking Covid-19 to the tune of "Come On Eileen",' he said.

'*Covid-19!*' I sang. '*Oh I uh-uh-uh-uh! Uh-uh-uh-uh-uh! So Covid-19! So Covid-19*'

'That's about as far as I got,' he said.

'I checked out Paul Hardcastle's "19". It's not a goer. Very few lyrics.'

'Yeah, I know,' he said.

'What about, "*When I was quarantined, it was a very good year . . .*" It's a Frank Sinatra song I think.'

'Oh yeah, that's good.'

Later, I checked. The song's called 'A Very Good Year', but there's only one verse about being seventeen and his other ages sound nothing like quarantine.

I spent most of the working day (all five hours of it) writing a treatment for a series looking back at my old programmes, featuring greatest-hits moments, hopefully tied together with some clever thesis which I haven't figured out yet. This is our solution to the making-programmes-without-meeting-people conundrum. We've been thinking for a couple of years of doing a one-hour retrospective. It was going to be pegged to my twenty-five years of making television anniversary, which was technically in 2019. Now, with gaping holes appearing in the TV schedule, the idea has been put on the front burner and expanded into a multipart extravaganza.

Mid-morning, on Instagram, I posted a couple of photos of a leek-based lasagne I'd made. I've been on a veggie lasagne jag, partly to relieve tension, mainly to have a pretext to lurk in the kitchen while drinking gin and tonic and listening to the radio. The creation of the food is a side effect. My American grandfather spent his twilight years in a shed next to his house on Cape Cod, hammering bits of wood together just to get some time to himself. He would use it all as fuel in the winter. My version is chopping an onion. In the afternoon, Nancy went to the Co-op. I sent a text to see if she could get the ingredients for a new lasagne recipe sent by a friend, involving roasted veg: **Courgettes, aubergines, peppers, basil, tomatoes**, I texted. She texted back a photo of a completely empty vegetable aisle.

I checked that Venice thing: 'Venetians say the water hasn't been this clear in sixty years.' Apparently it's cobblers. It's just that there's less traffic on the canals, so the sediment is staying on the bottom.

10.45 p.m.
I just came up to bed. The boys were printing out their schedules. Enjoying the change of routine.

Friday 20 March

They have actioned the lockdown plan. We are no longer allowed to go to pubs, restaurants, theatres, gyms. Everyone other than key workers is encouraged to stay home and in public places we have to stay two metres apart. The total UK death toll so far is 184. In Italy they reported 627 people dead just today.

The two big boys had their first day at home. For their remote learning, they both need laptops, which Arthur has but Jack doesn't. I'd dug up an old Powerbook which is clogged up with malware and system conflicts and booked it in for a repair at a place in Hampstead above a Porsche dealership, Apple stores all being closed.

'I have asthma, right,' said the repairman on the phone, who was from Wolverhampton. 'So I'm high risk. When you come, I'm going to give you a single-use face mask. I'll drop it through the window as you stand outside. I'll then give you antibacterial spray for your hands. I don't mean to be unfriendly but I can't take any risks.'

In the afternoon I picked Ray up from school. On the way back he said, 'Do you know if a bullet goes into your brain you die?'

'Yes. That's right. Because do you know what death means?' I asked.

'You go to heaven?' he said.

'Er, kind of. I meant more what it means in your body. Something happens to it.'

'You close your eyes?' He quickly thought better of this. 'No, because that can be sleeping. You go floppy?'

'It just means oxygen is no longer reaching your brain. So that's why you could die from being shot in the brain or the heart.'

No comment from Ray, and I remembered I was talking to a five-year-old.

They are now saying it may be a year until we are back to normal.

Do I actually believe this? I'm not sure. Nothing feels quite real. I'd like to think that I am, in a mature way, resigned to a situation that is wholly outside my control. But it's just as possible that I'm losing my shit and I just haven't noticed yet.

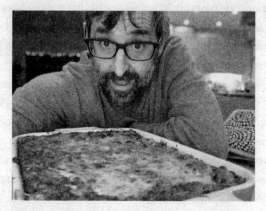

The first of many lockdown vegetarian lasagnes.

Saturday 21 March

The lockdown is fully in place now. As a weekend outing we'd been hoping to go to the grounds of Cliveden, the stately home west of London that used to belong to the Astors. But the National Trust has closed it. In the end we went to Hampstead Heath and met up with some friends and their children – bashing elbows together, no contact, wry remarks about 'social distancing!' and 'two metres!' Within fifteen minutes, the boys – five of them – were bundling on the ground and Arthur was complaining that someone had bitten him.

The park cafe was closed but other than that it was busy and the only difference from a normal visit was that all the conversations when you got close seemed to be about the virus.

Eco-Photographer Friend was saying: 'I really think this virus is showing what the world can do in terms of cooperation. The top, top scientists are putting aside their differences and going to work on this thing.'

Advertising Friend, less idealistic, or maybe just realistic, replied: 'Are you serious? I think that's the exact opposite of what's happening.'

'No, they're really pooling their research efforts. It's a model for how we can work together.'

'*Time out*. Mate. China sat on the fact that there was an outbreak for *five weeks*. Told no one. Meanwhile, people are coming and going. They imprisoned the main whistleblower.'

I was earwigging while throwing a frisbee back and forth with Ray.

A small child arrived, maybe two or three years old, with copper ringlets of hair and a dummy attached to a ribbon. She/he was seemingly without provenance, like a Russian bot looking to infect us, wordless, calm and rather adorable, wandering up and trying to take our football away. Who was the parent? Off in the distance, fifty metres away, was a glamorous but oblivious young woman, sitting down in spray-on jeans, wiping mud from her boot with a seemingly endless supply of wet wipes. Only the pushchair she had with her suggested the child might be hers. Ten or fifteen minutes later, the child had wandered away from us towards a lake, albeit a fenced-off one. The glamorous woman roused herself, calling wanly in a faint Russian accent, 'Angelika!' or possibly, 'Angeliko!'

The toddler ignored the call, still heading towards the water, until disaster struck in the form of a patch of mud, where he or she slipped and now lay crying. The woman wandered down, with no sense of urgency, and then tried to prevail on bystanders to go and get the child for her, so she didn't have to get dirty.

Another woman, a stranger, picked the child up. I was too far away to hear but she seemed to remonstrate with the distracted woman as she handed the child over. When we left, the mother was taking out more wipes and mopping away a tiny amount of dirt from the child, who looked on without emotion. What was wrong with the woman, I wondered. How was it possible that her child was so calm and well-adjusted? Was it possible that having a bonkers parent instilled tolerance and forbearance in a child? Was *that* where I was going wrong?

Sunday 22 March

An item on Radio 4 about woodcocks and their feathers and seeing them in the wild. Anything not about the virus feels hopelessly irrelevant. I switched to 5 Live. They were saying that in Italy the total number of deaths now stands at 5,000. Whenever a pundit or a reporter spoke, you could hear from the acoustics that they were calling in from their homes. Everything had a muffled bunker feel, but they carried on as if it was normal. 'I'm at home, where I've self-isolated.'

There are mutterings that Boris Johnson left the lockdown too late and should have closed parks earlier. I flashed back to our kids wrestling and biting each other on Hampstead Heath.

The prevailing strange emotion, which one hesitates to acknowledge, is the shameful excitement at living in an apocalyptic scenario. A movie has come to life and engulfed us. Aliens, zombies, paranormal events – the tropes of Hollywood – have become our day-to-day reality and I still get a little pulse of excitement when I see the masks and the signs and the news bulletins. But then I was cycling back from the computer repair shop listening to the *This American Life* podcast and at the end Ira Glass, the host, said that when timing your hand-washing, instead of singing 'Happy Birthday' twice you can also sing one whole chorus of 'Stayin' Alive'. And then they played it, the Bee Gees singing in shimmering falsetto, and for a moment I was ambushed by a strange sensation and I wondered what I was feeling and was I about to cry?

Monday 23 March

First weekday with all three children at home.

In order to simulate the normal morning commute, and to get some exercise, I went for a cycle around the local area, down Sidmouth Parade, past Edward VII Park, to the top of Scrubs Lane and back. The streets were empty, very few cars on the road or people out walking. An eerie sense of quiet that was at the same time calming: a feeling that we are *doing this*, we are trusting the plan and locking ourselves away, and maybe it will all be over relatively soon, and in any event there is something to appreciate in the peace and quiet and the absence of the usual urban aggro.

Jack, commencing homeschooling, wanted his phone in his room. I said no, and asked for him to hand it over, which he declined to do, which in turn led to a meltdown, mainly by me. He had hidden the phone somewhere down the side of his chair or his desk, I wasn't sure exactly where, and I had a strong urge to ferret it out and confiscate it but I also didn't want to become the desperate man reduced to hunting for his son's phone, screaming, 'WHERE IS IT? GIVE IT TO ME!!' I walked away, not sure if I'd caved in or seen reason. The kids have so little contact with their friends, I told myself it was fair enough to let them text or speak on their devices – the lockdown equivalent of chatting in class. Arthur, meanwhile, is largely getting on with his work, perhaps even enjoying the new rules and the sense of occasion.

Ray wanted to wear his school uniform, even though he wasn't going to school, which was faintly heartbreaking. We did some bouncing ball games in the hall, and then some 'phonics'. 'Cah and Hah are special friends and when they are together they make a "Cha" sound.' Then he helped me mow the lawn. I hope he wasn't too disappointed. Something tells me he had high hopes for 'homeschool' with Mr Louis and Ms Nancy and I'm not sure we met them.

From 1.30 p.m. to 3 p.m. Nancy and I traded off. I worked and she did activities with Ray. Then I came down to find Nancy had arranged with a neighbour that I was going to take her two children, aged eight and eleven, to the park. I was dubious but felt cornered, and took them but spent the entire outing making curt demands: 'Move away from each other! MOVE AWAY!'

When I got home, I said to Nancy, 'Well, if they didn't have Covid before they've got it now . . . You know we can't be doing that. Kids don't understand social distancing.'

Then, I said: 'Where's Arthur?'

'He's out with friends.'

'Nancy, have you not been listening to the news or reading Twitter? We're supposed to be locked down!'

'I was on a conference call and he just came in and said he was going out.'

'You've heard about the pandemic? The one that's killing tons of people?'

She huffed and rolled her eyes, which was probably only what the comment deserved, and just then Arthur sauntered out of his bedroom, where he'd been the whole time.

Around 8.30, Boris made an announcement that we were locking-down further. Only allowed out once a day for exercise and essential shopping.

I spent the evening making a BBC Food vegetarian lasagne, based mainly on courgettes and peppers, while listening to a BBC podcast about Alex Salmond's sexual assault trial. This is what passes for recreation in these times.

Tuesday 24 March

Again comes the question of what we now do as work. Some part of me is struggling to adjust. We've been discussing the possibility of me hosting a podcast. An interview series of some kind in which I speak to people remotely, via the Internet, the theory being that a higher calibre of celebrity guest may now be available, since everyone is locked down, their projects on hold. Someone at Radio 4 has been in touch – they're keen. Podcasting is something people have suggested I do over the last couple of years. I've resisted, feeling the market may be saturated. I suspect there are more podcasts than there are people to listen to them at this point.

The idea of a podcast has me worried – the possibility of failure, the prospect of working with famous and talented people who I may be in awe of and whose time is precious, for whom the idea of a long-form conversation with a podcast noob is the last thing they feel like participating in. What I've always enjoyed about my work is the promise of invisibility, being immersed in worlds where I'm unknown, in lives utterly different from my own, a captive of their mindset and their lifestyle. With a podcast, does that still apply? It seems almost the opposite: me on the main stage, having to perform. But the company needs to keep busy, we have salaries to justify, and I also recognize my anxiety as an old antagonist, a saboteur intent on derailing my efforts. The fear isn't necessarily founded in anything real, and in fact may be a sign that I should go ahead.

Still, out of puckishness, and as a way of asserting control, I've been suggesting left-field names as guests to Radio 4, like the ultra-right-wing ex-MP Harvey Proctor, who left parliament over a low-level sex scandal and was later hounded and defamed on wholly false allegations of being involved in paedophilia and satanic ritual abuse.

'I think he'd be a great interview,' I said to Arron. 'His life was nearly destroyed. Can you imagine? Being accused of dismembering small children?'

'I ran it by Radio 4. They didn't say no but I don't think he'd be their top choice. They were wondering about Daniel Craig.'

'The Bond actor? I don't know much about him.'

'Apparently they have a line to him.'

'And that's a reason to do him?'

Earlier in the day, Nancy had mentioned that Joe Wicks, the floppy-haired fitness guru, has started a live daily work-out session, streaming it on his YouTube channel. At five to nine, we balanced the laptop on a sofa next to the kitchen and the five of us stood in a row, each on a little patch of carpet, and went through the exercises: running on the spot, squats, lunges, mountain climbers, all in thirty-second increments with thirty-second rests.

Ray joined in, doing very rough interpretations of the movements. I felt better afterwards and reflected that if nothing else lockdown might be a chance to get fit. I've sometimes daydreamed about spending a month living at a spa getting ripped and limber. Maybe this was going to be a kind of suboptimal fulfilment of that fantasy.

In the afternoon, I had an hour and a half to work on a treatment for a documentary series we are pitching about the case of Jeremy Bamber, who in 1986, as a young man, was convicted of killing his sister, their parents, and her two young children at the family farmhouse in Essex. Bamber is unique among prisoners serving whole-life terms in the UK in having always maintained his innocence. His claim is that his sister killed the family – she had a documented history of serious mental illness – then turned the gun on herself. Nancy has been driving the idea for several months with a colleague at Mindhouse called Flo – there's a chance we may get an interview with Bamber via his team of supporters, who are campaigning for his release.

At 3.30, Nancy came to tell me I was back on Ray duty. We got into a stupid argument about the work I'd been doing. We were both tense, cabin-crazy, frustrated about the inability to get anything done, and the uncertainty hanging over the future of the business. I was carrying Ray downstairs as we shouted back and forth.

'I can't believe you're tearing a strip off me for trying to help!' I said. 'Fine! You do it!' 'I don't even want to do it! You told me to take it over!'

Ray hasn't heard us argue much, and while he didn't complain or cry he did begin chanting, not loudly but insistently, almost to himself, 'Brrrr. No! Brrrrrr. No! Brrrrr. No!' – in a kind of imprecation to make us stop.

Number of deaths in the UK stands at 422 as of noon yesterday. Globally, 18,200.

Wednesday 25 March

Many are speculating on whether the lockdown will strain relationships. I bumped into a divorced neighbour making a visit to his old home.

'I want to invent an app. Get divorced quick. You just push the button. Wife gets a text. "You're divorced."'

'Interesting idea,' I said.

'Tell you what, though,' he went on. 'What worries me. You're going to get a whole load of divorces and at the same time a baby boom.'

'OK,' I said. 'Yeah.'

But I was thinking: *Baby boom. Seriously?* Because nothing puts lead in your pencil like being locked down in a house with your kids 24/7, loading and unloading the dishwasher.

Thursday 26 March

'Please, Dad, can you imitate?' Ray said, meaning 'commentate' on a trampoline game that involves him bouncing and dodging balls. I put on my 'radio voice'.

'Here we are at the Willesden Stadium for this latest event in the Tramp-o-lympics. And our tenacious competitor Ray Theroux is about to get started.'

'Can you be on my teen?' Ray said, meaning 'team'.

I got inside and bounced with him. Afterwards I lay on my back with his head on my chest. He said, 'I can hear your heart beep.'

It was in the news today that Prince Charles tested positive. I wonder, does so many rich and famous people having it suggest there are many more undiscovered positives among the less rich and less famous who don't have access to tests?

On the plus side, a tweet I sent the other day – 'My hands are so dry they feel like they belong to someone else' – has had 20,000 likes.

Friday 27 March

We've been watching a new seven-part Netflix series about American big-cat owners, called *Tiger King*.

The main character is Joe Exotic, a colourful Oklahoma zoo owner with 200 tigers, several body piercings, two lovers, and one mullet. His sworn enemy is an animal rights activist named Carole Baskin, who runs a sanctuary for rescued animals and has a penchant for wearing floaty animal print frocks and headdresses. There are assorted other supporting players, all weird in different ways, sexually unconventional, drug-ravaged, narcissistic, obsessive or dissolute. The series is big and brash, with explosions and slow-motion sequences of the main players looking meaningfully into camera. It tracks Joe's mounting obsession with Carole, culminating in his attempt to have her killed and his resulting federal prosecution in a murder-for-hire case.

Launched at any time, *Tiger King* would have been a hit, I'm sure, but in Covid World, with very little to distract us from the distressing news and people going out of their minds with boredom, it is showing signs of becoming a seismic pop cultural phenomenon, the Internet going crazy as fans obsess over whether Carole Baskin might have murdered her husband, and celebrities dressing up as characters. There are memes and clips showing Joe's catchphrase – 'That bitch Carole Baskin' – and of him saying, after an employee gets his arm bitten off by a tiger, 'I am never gonna financially recover from this.' Among other things, it is a testament to the power of social media. It is perhaps the media analogue to the pandemic itself, literally going viral, even faster than Covid, because unlike a physical virus, it doesn't require passenger planes and body fluids to spread but can travel the digital ether into sixty million homes simultaneously, via the miracle of Netflix.

Making it all the stranger for me is that I know Joe, and several other of the characters, having made my own documentary about big-cat owners in 2011, *America's Most Dangerous Pets*. I know Joe, I know his ex-husband John Finlay, I know his right-hand man John Reinke. I know his friend Tim Stark. I don't know Carole but I think we had some email contact with her back in the day.

I also know a couple of the people involved in making the series. I doff my cap to their execution of the project, the many laughs and the high-octane storytelling that has captivated the world. Once or twice I've been asked by people who know about my history with Joe whether I feel chagrined at having seemingly narrowly missed out on being part of possibly the biggest documentary hit of all time. I look into my heart and I say, as honestly as I can, no. The truth is, I was never in a position to make *Tiger King*. The federal case that provides the spine of the series was still far in the future when I filmed in 2011. If anything, I'm mainly pleased that I can claim some kind of foresight in taking an interest in Joe's story so many years ahead of the curve – recognizing as I did that it's pretty weird for so many Americans to be keeping majestic animals like tigers, lions and bears in captivity in large numbers – and I'm grateful that some people have noticed that I planted a small flag in the terrain.

However, it *is* slightly odd to find out that when throwing a barbecue for me and the crew back in 2011, Joe almost certainly used expired meat donated by Walmart that was intended for the animals.

Saturday 28 March

Ray and I were doing the food shop.

Outside Sainsbury's Willesden in the parking lot: a long snaking line of people all two metres apart, some of them in masks. We drove to Blue Mountain in Harlesden. It was closed. We tried the Co-op in Queen's Park, which was open. No lemons and limes, no carrots, no grapes, fruit and veg thin in general. No pasta, of course, and not many tinned goods, but other than that it was reasonably well stocked. We moved on to the Sainsbury's Local, where I bought a couple of top-up items, and then finally a retailer of insanely over-priced organic food, which brought us to five supermarkets.

News came through yesterday that Boris Johnson has the virus. Health Minister Matt Hancock has it too and Chief Medical Adviser Chris Whitty. VIP cases supplying further evidence that there may be thousands of others with Covid who just haven't been tested yet.

Today, Saturday, is not much different from a weekday. Restless-ness from the troops because they 'only' get an hour of PlayStation time a day. This is seen as a human rights violation that should be litigated at The Hague. We are trying to incentivize the kids to do chores, to earn their PS times, which is also viewed as extreme and tyrannical. Today, Jack swept the stairs and cleaned two pairs of shoes, and Arthur cleared out a cupboard. Then Nancy said we'd be going for a walk in some woods after lunch, location TBD, to blow off some steam. Jack was not a fan of the concept. He wanted to get on the PS.

'NOOO! I'M NOT GOING!!!'

'Jack, you'd think you'd been told you're about to have some teeth pulled!'

Museum, gallery, woods, adventure – all these words are

triggers. 'I'm not going to some dumb weirdo woods to look at some stupid trees!'

Total Covid deaths in UK are now 1,019. Which is up 260. People keep saying, in emails and small talk, 'Strange times!' The phrase is now rote. I feel like there should be something else to say but I don't know what it is.

At the same time, at some dark and unacknowledged level, I seem to have a fear of things returning to normal. From Hawaii, where he lives, my dad sent a message saying how clarifying and salutary he finds the pandemic. Exposing leaders for who they are. Forcing people to think and re-evaluate and recognize their lack of control over events and maybe their own irrelevance. And it is true, too, that amid the panic and sadness is a strange feeling of privilege to be alive at a historic moment. That I, who was spared the scourge of world wars and famines, have lived to see a world upended by pestilence.

Maybe that's what my dad was talking about. I wonder if, having already sunk so much fear and anxiety into what is happening, I am now invested in the idea of a disaster, like a small child smashing his own toys to vindicate his rage and the righteousness of his feelings of being victimized. Or maybe it's something simpler – the sense of upheaval produces a sense of perspective on the small anxieties that ordinarily assail us. Like riots or extreme weather – the chaos lifts some sense of responsibility from us. The normal rules don't apply, we have an excuse when things don't work out, for our myriad failures, and we can take a breath, enjoy the sense of proportion provided by a far greater calamity, and relax a little bit.

Yesterday we ate some leftovers for lunch, including a ratatouille. 'Ratatouille is just BTEC Bolognese,' I said to Jack.

'Exactly,' he said.

Sunday 29 March

Major mutiny among the troops due to alleged tyrannical abuses by army high command. Nancy had words with them. Jack was suggesting that there should be *no* regulation of PlayStation time. His theory, working off the old adage about chocolate factory workers growing sick of chocolate, was that if they had unlimited access to the console they would go on it *less* because it would lose its cachet.

'But kids don't always get bored of PlayStation,' I said. 'There are people who stay on it ten or twelve hours a day. They wear nappies and don't even stop playing to take a poop.'

'You've been watching *Dr Phil*,' Jack said.

'I don't watch *Dr Phil*,' I protested.

Their compromise suggestion – that they should go on for two shifts of three hours each, nine to twelve and one to four – was roundly and robustly rejected by top brass.

I felt under the weather today. All day on lockdown. Didn't go out. Ray pleading with me to go on the trampoline with him and me just not feeling I could face it.

Tuesday 31 March

Full-on meltdown at lunch, this time by me.

We had all woken up late, at 8.45. I had a call with Arron and Paul, the producer of the podcast, which is moving ahead. Then Nancy came back from a supermarket run to say there was no fruit and no vegetables and no milk. Late morning, I went out with Jack on a bicycle trip to a local shop, Khan Halal Butchers, off Willesden High Road. Inside they had everything you could dream of. Tinned tomatoes. Apples. Tamarind paste.

'Auntie, please, two metres,' the manager said to a heavyset woman in a mask. She giggled. 'You laugh but it is serious,' he continued.

I wobbled home on the bike with the groceries in bags hanging from the handlebars.

At lunchtime I put out a variety of options – leftover lentil soup, vegetarian lasagne, chicken and lemon pasta. Ray didn't want to eat his chicken.

'Do the giant game!' he said.

'OK, if you'll eat your peas.'

'Do the giant game for the chicken.'

'I don't want to do the giant game for chicken. It's only for peas.'

'Please!'

The giant game involves me pretending to be a giant falling asleep, while Ray eats the food on his plate. I then wake up enraged to find 'my' food gone. It's supposed to incentivize him to eat food he might not normally eat. Like vegetables. Chicken doesn't usually count. But I found myself relenting.

'DON'T EAT MY CHICKEN!!' I yelled. 'DON'T TOUCH MY CHICKEN!!!'

Ray giggled, happy now, but the volume and intensity of my speech told me I was close to the edge of a manic episode, a cocktail of overexcitement and anger. It's a state I sometimes get into when I'm stressed or underslept or over-tweaked. I closed my eyes, pretending to sleep. Ray ate a little chicken.

Nancy came in, took a piece of bread, and ambled over. Crumbs were dropping on the floor.

'You're dropping crumbs,' I said, annoyed.

'What's got into you?' she said.

'Nothing, I'm just telling you. You're dropping crumbs. You might need a plate?'

'I don't know what's up with you but you are turning into monster mode.'

'OK, so, you are the one shouting at ME right now,' I said.

Ray had started hitting me, which is a thing he does at the moment. The hits are more symbolic than intended to hurt but on this occasion I turned on him and shouted, 'STOP HITTING ME YOU'RE HURTING ME!' and he burst into tears. And it more or less went from there, Nancy picked Ray up in her arms, 'What is WRONG with you?' etc, the kids fell silent, which was probably the worst part, their lack of reaction, and then Arthur and Jack left the room, ushering Ray before them. And then I was on my own in the kitchen for an hour or so, Arthur having taken it upon himself to entertain Ray. They snuck in for some sweets, giggling, then ran off again, staying away.

One part of me felt ashamed and remorseful, another part was thinking, *Oh, so if you completely lose your shit, you are left alone and everything is recalibrated, so maybe that is a good result?* Jack came down and hugged me after about forty-five minutes. Then an hour or two later it was mostly back to normal. At 5.30 or so I ordered a couple of Domino's pizzas. It was two for one Tuesdays, so in a way it all worked out.

More than 3,000 total deaths in the US. They may mount as high as 100,000, they say. Is that possible? In the evening, watched last episode of *Tiger King*.

April 2020

PODCAST NOOB

Sunday 5 April

'Should Veronica come? She's texted,' Nancy said.

Veronica is the cleaner.

'No,' I said. 'We should pay her, but it's still too early.'

This was at eight in the morning. An hour or so later, there was a ring at the door. It was Veronica, wearing a face mask, and looking emotional.

'I not get message,' she said. 'I at home, miss people.'

What's she doing here? Nancy said with her eyes and her eyebrows.

'She's lonely,' I hissed. 'She's missing people. She seemed near tears. What am I supposed to say? Hop it? Can't come in?'

'Well, I think we should ask her to leave early. She's not supposed to be here.'

'Sure, I'll just say we don't need downstairs doing.'

Veronica moved around the house, cleaning as usual, except that we and the three kids were all around and the world was dying of Covid-19.

Late morning, she came downstairs and stood in the kitchen with the air of someone with something to announce. 'You are my angels.' Then, in her faltering English, she said that before she arrived in the UK, back in Brazil, she'd seen a documentary I'd made about children with autism and families struggling to cope. She said she has two children with autism – one of the reasons she's here is to send money back to them. She'd never mentioned it before, she said, but the programme had helped her family understand what she was going through. Her little speech was so touching and unexpected that I became focused on meeting it with an equivalent gesture of appreciation. In a robot-like way I determined it was – *doot doot doot* – an *emotional moment* – *doot*

doot doot – and my fellow-human-analysis circuits suggested some physical reassurance might be required. *Initiate hug protocol.* I moved towards her with deliberateness, signalling my intention, so as to avoid misunderstandings and therefore awkwardness, my arms open, as she looked back at me with horror, recognizing that I was about to break the prime directive of Covid World: *not to touch. Doot doot doot! Abort! Abort!* I apologized and retreated.

Global cases have reached 1 million. UK cases, 38,168 with 3605 total deaths.

Monday 6 April

News today that Boris Johnson has been admitted to hospital. Socialist Nancy, smelling a rat, said, 'Are they making it sound worse than it is, for sympathy? Or do you think it's more serious than they're letting on, and they're hiding it, to prevent panic?'

By the end of the day – around 8 p.m. – word came that he was in ICU. We watched *News at Ten*, for the first time in years. Both Arthur and Jack were on their phones. Me thinking, *You'll never see anything quite like this again.* There was a report from University College Hospital. Reporter wearing face mask and visor. Doctor near tears talking about his family. They had an interview with a bus driver in the hospital – several bus drivers have died, exposed to passengers as they board. More than 5,000 fatalities in the UK now. 'Mainly high blood pressure, diabetic,' the doctor said, 'but some healthy younger people.'

Thursday 9 April

A pizza oven has arrived. A company reached out via Instagram to ask if I was interested in one, having, I assume, seen some of my posts about making vegetarian lasagnes. I assembled it in the garden, by which I mean, I screwed on the legs and a little metal chimney. It's stainless steel and has a small hatch where you load on twigs and sticks, like an engineer on a steam train. Apparently, the key to great pizza crust is very high heat. This oven is designed to withstand 400°C – it came with a laser gun to check the temperature – and it cooks the dough in about a minute and a half, creating the little black scorch marks, or 'leopard spotting', which are the hallmark of the superior crust. It combines two distinct guilty pleasures, both close to my heart: gastronomy and pyromania.

In the evening I watched a special episode of *Horizon* with Arthur and Jack, dedicated to the pandemic. On the question of whether the virus arose as a result of someone eating a bat or a pangolin, it seemed to be saying that someone had eaten a pangolin that had eaten a bat. And that bats are incubators of viruses because of their status as flying mammals that live in cities. Cities of bats. I know, it wasn't very clear. The other takeaway was that bacteria can, apparently, catch viruses.

'Maybe e-coli will catch ebola,' Arthur said.

Friday 10 April

Easter Friday, and also my dad's birthday. I belatedly ordered him a *Big Lebowski* themed T-shirt off Amazon – the Dude as Vitruvian man, holding bowling ball, etc. I kind of wanted to send him the one that said, 'Hey, careful, there's a beverage here!' in big lettering, but worried it was maybe too brash for a seventy-nine-year-old *homme de lettres* to comfortably be seen in.

In the afternoon, I retreated to the spare bedroom on the top floor and recorded a chat with Jon Ronson for the new podcast. My inaugural guest, and he delivered urbane repartee and acute cultural observation in well-proportioned quantities. He lives in upstate New York, in the woods somewhere, and I had the sense the pandemic had not massively altered his routines. We talked about our rivalry in the nineties and early oughts. He is a couple of years older than me, and his early TV series *The Ronson Mission* had been an influence on my first series, *Weird Weekends*. Later he'd confessed to profound feelings of envy about the success of *Weird Weekends*. We covered similar subjects in our work – mental illness and unconventional lifestyles – and years later he'd commented in print, 'I sometimes think that Louis and I are like conjoined twins and that one of us must die so that the other can live.'

Jon sees a lot of positives in the response to the pandemic: people largely *not* turning on one another in feral packs. He has been open about having a diagnosed anxiety disorder and said his symptoms have been alleviated by the advent of the Covid phenomenon. In his view, a tendency to catastrophize can serve as helpful preparation for an actual catastrophe.

We also talked about the various conspiracy theories that have been thriving in lockdown, many of them perpetuated by his one-time subjects, former Coventry goalkeeper David Icke and shouty

American radio host Alex Jones. According to the theories, Covid is bioengineered, part of a plan to implement global control through chipping – 'plandemic' is the phrase – or possibly it is a reaction to 5G masts or it's spread in populations with immune systems weakened by 5G. Icke's second act as a paranoid prophet of the New Age has turned out to have legs no one could have imagined when he first announced himself as the second coming of Christ on an episode of *Wogan* in 1991. Some of those under his influence have gone about burning down phone masts. A couple of days ago YouTube and Facebook took down videos linking 5G and Covid, an act of suppression which briefly gave the idea more traction. A textbook case of the Streisand Effect: attempts by the singer to remove aerial photos of her home from the Internet in 2003 inadvertently led to more people viewing the photos.

This led to a conversation about Jon's view of deplatforming and the extent to which free speech should be curbed on social media. He said, whatever one's views of whether it's ethical, it does work. People can be muzzled. He was recently denounced by Alex Jones, and whereas in former times Jon might have expected to be trolled by Jones's outriders, now that Jones has no platform on Facebook or Twitter, the attacks were barely noticeable.

The question of which views get to be heard on social media is now, in the Coronaverse, high stakes. There are weird graphs on Twitter from right-wing columnist Peter Hitchens and Dilbert cartoonist Scott Adams and American novelist Walter Kirn suggesting that 'normal' pneumonia deaths are being totted up as Covid deaths. Another article suggests that Neil Ferguson, the UK health guru, has form for overreaching during viral outbreaks, killing too many animals during the foot-and-mouth scare, for example, and that the lockdown is unnecessary.

One suspects there would be more Covid unrest except for the long spell of beautiful weather buoying up people's spirits. Boris apparently out of ICU but still in hospital.

Some debate about how long the lockdown will last. Weeks? Months? Will the children go back for summer term or not? At the moment it seems unlikely. So, the bad part is, the economy is collapsing, thousands are dying and millions are in distress. But the good part is, I can go out in my pyjamas.

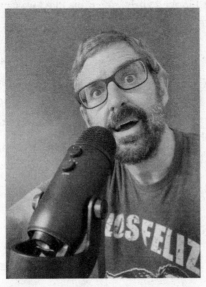

The Dame Vera Lynn of Lockdown Podcasting™ in action.

Saturday 11 April

Another day of at-homeness. Mid-afternoon I did a shop at the local Co-op. Nancy warned me there was now social pressure to wear a mask. Not having a mask, I brought a scarf and wrapped it around my face. In my slippers and light cotton outerwear I was conscious that I looked fairly ludicrous, like I was auditioning for a remake of *Lawrence of Arabia* in which he leads an independence movement seeking to liberate the shops in Sidmouth Parade. Also, I kept getting recognized – 'kept' as in it happened twice – by people who'd seen my *Dangerous Pets* programme, which recently re-aired on BBC Two in the wake of the *Tiger King* phenomenon. Did they imagine I was swaddled up like Katharine Hepburn, trying – with maximum visibility – to avoid attention?

Monday 13 April

Easter Monday. In Lockdown Land, with nowhere to go, the idea of holidays is essentially meaningless, and so we had a catch-up about the podcast – me and the small team we've assembled, all of us on Zoom. The chat lasted about an hour, some of it about possible titles. Radio 4 has suggested 'Grounded', which Arron isn't sold on.

'I spoke to a friend who works in marketing and she wasn't a fan,' he said.

I was neutral on it. Other ideas were 'Locked Down', 'Lock-In', 'Therouxpy', 'PandeMOANium'. 'I don't think "Grounded" is too bad,' I said at the end, 'but we can keep thinking.'

Afterwards I came downstairs to the first floor with a spring in my step, feeling like I'd done a day's work. I spotted an overflowing basket of clean clothes.

'Shall I put the laundry away?'

'Not if it's going to take you an hour,' Nancy said, a little unkindly. She was midway through doing a cull of Ray's basket of fancy dress. Nancy is not in a good mood due to grief over the revelation that Jeremy Corbyn's enemies in the Labour Party actively undermined the party's 2017 election campaign, so they could get rid of him.

Wednesday 15 April

Yes, I am drinking too much, but am I drinking much more than the too-much I normally drink? Hard to say.

Alcohol – the non-board-certified Dr Ink – has been my mental health practitioner of choice going back twenty-five years or more. My prescription has remained fairly consistent: a gin and tonic or two per night, around six o'clock, followed up with several glasses of red wine. Side effects include slurring, thinking I'm funnier than I actually am, sometimes dancing, followed by mild grumpiness in the morning.

The drinking has, naturally, been accompanied by a low-level concern that I'm overdoing it, and occasional half-hearted attempts to cut back a bit.

A couple of weeks before lockdown I arrived at work hungover, and seemingly aware my kidneys hurt, or maybe my liver, or anyway some organ which I supposed had something to do with metabolizing alcohol. I called the doctor to get tested. I wasn't sure what the test might be, I just imagined there must be some diagnostic process that would reveal any inner damage and that might induce her to say: *Uh-oh, the jig is up, party's over gramps, time to take it easy, even if it's just two nights off a week, slow down.*

I got the tests. A few days later they came back, and the verdict was: fine. Nothing to worry about, keep going. I was almost slightly disappointed.

So, the routine continues, possibly with a slight uptick in intake, due to not going out, and maybe anxiety.

On Monday night Nancy accused me of being drunk. But I think she was drunk, so I'm not sure it counts. Tonight she took it further and accused me of drinking too much of the Robinsons 'Real Fruit in Every Drop – Summer Fruits' cordial.

'You are reaching,' I said. 'You're lumping together me drinking too much gin with me drinking the Robinsons fruit drink?'

'It's the kids'!'

'I'll buy some more.'

'That's not the point.'

'Do you know how you sound?'

'You're drinking it *as mixer*. That's why you're drinking it. So it's related.'

Some other countries are loosening lockdown. Danish primary schools are reopening. Spanish schools. Here in the UK, lockdown continues and we are on course to be the worst hit in Europe. So far, 130,000 deaths worldwide, and 2 million cases. A dawning realization that Covid-19 is not going away and we will all have to get used to a different way of living, though what exactly it will be like is unclear.

Meanwhile an email from Advertising Friend. He sometimes sends jokes. 'Just heard that there will be a round of applause for couriers and delivery drivers,' he writes. 'It will be sometime between 9 a.m. and 5 p.m. tomorrow.'

Sunday 19 April

Just about recovered from an indoor solo Saturday night sesh that slightly got away from me.

It started innocently enough, with Nancy watching television and me listening to hip hop and reggae on the Google Home in the kitchen. Notionally, I was compiling tracks for a playlist for BBC Sounds that would cross-promote the podcast. One track led to another. 'Fade Away' by New Age Steppers, which I was listening to because Boy George, who I'd interviewed for the podcast, had mentioned that the lead singer Ari Up was a style icon and influence on his look in the early eighties. This led me to check out the original of 'Fade Away', by Junior Byles, and then 'Silly Games' by Janet Kay, which I read is an example of the 'Willesden Sound'. This was exciting, since we live in Willesden. Then I put on Conor Oberst and Monsters of Folk and Brit Daniel, the lead singer of the Texas group Spoon. I was drinking Kentucky bourbon mixed with ruby grapefruit breakfast juice, while ferrying in glasses of Prosecco to Nancy piously, as though I was being abstemious and considerate. 'No, *you* have the last of the Prosecco.' Suddenly it was one thirty and I realized I needed to turn in. I was 'on Ray duty' – which means going in with him when required.

The next morning he was up around 7.30. I carried him downstairs. I'd only slept five or six hours and was feeling as though Junior Byles had taken a shit in my head.

'Shall we watch some T V? What do you want to watch?'

'I want to watch the one with the devil,' Ray said.

I remembered that I'd ill-advisedly allowed him to watch the first half of *Hellboy*. It is not in fact an 18, but a 15. Ray is five. Sigh. Nancy had not been in favour. I put it on and lay back on the sofa trying to doze. Ray was climbing over me, then attempting to get comfortable in a way that involved using my body as a kind of daybed. I peered at the screen. Hellboy was wisecracking and delivering sassy putdowns in a New York accent. He was a take-no-shit devil creature with big sawn-off horns and nothing fazed him. Then a creepy ghost woman appeared. Even Hellboy seemed worried by her. Then an old witch-lady, with one eye, who was writhing and doing backflips.

'She's a serial killer,' the five-year-old says.

'Mmm. How do you know about serial killers?'

'That museum. Remember?'

I recalled a visit to Hastings last year and a museum of crime – it had seemed innocent enough at the time: exhibits about gangsters and a woman who kept adopting small infants in apparent acts of charity, soliciting donations, and then murdering the children. Yeah. Come to think of it, maybe that was a weird move, taking him. Back in the present, the weird witch-lady opened a door to a room full of what appeared to be murdered children hanging on ropes.

'OK, that's enough of that,' I said, switching it off. Ray wailed and shouted, but even hungover underslept Louis at 7.30 a.m. has some standards, and I found something on TV that didn't involve mass infant death. In the afternoon, I paid ten pounds to download *101 Dalmatians*, the Disney original, which he watched while I had the most enriching ten- or fifteen-minute sleep of recent times.

Tuesday 21 April

Lockdown in UK extended another three weeks. Confirmed toll in Europe has passed 1 million with 100,000 deaths. In America, Trump is encouraging people to break the lockdown and oil now has a negative price due to storage facilities being full up. That has to be a good thing, right? Undermine the Saudi regime by not needing any of their oil?

In the afternoon I was trying to work – listening to the interview I did with Jon Ronson for the podcast – while also Ray-sitting. He was getting frustrated, not enjoying the games he'd downloaded, while I was feeling stressed about aspects of the podcast – Paul, the producer, has edited it down to an hour plus change, but I worry my questions are rambling and unfocused, and that I failed to impose enough of a shape on the chat, and specifically that I didn't at any point near the beginning tee up a thesis. 'Why I'm interested in you, Jon . . .' kind of thing. As I was thinking this, and the frustration and self-recrimination was kicking in, every minute or two Ray would cry or scream or become exasperated about wanting to download an app involving a red ball but he doesn't know what it's called, and my stress levels would spike into the red, with an alarming surge of anger and impatience. The combination of urgent work pressure and a child unhappy with my iPhone turns out to be surprisingly incapacitating and should maybe be considered for use at black sites by the CIA as an alternative to 'enhanced interrogation'.

Kids went back to school today. Virtual school that is. 'End of Easter Holidays.' In inverted commas.

Wednesday 22 April

A day of publicity to promote *Grounded with Louis Theroux* (we went with the title) which is launching in a few days. There is such a shortfall of product due to lockdown that it feels as though anything new is garlanded with extra attention. It's said I may go on *Graham Norton*. To promote a podcast on a TV chat show seems a reversal of the natural order of things – like a horse riding a man.

As a result of the over-full schedule of remote interviews, I missed my first Joe Wicks workout since he began his live sessions. I mentioned this during a chat with LADbible, and talked about my life-changing commitment to the Gospel of Wicks, and then heard myself launch into a very camp and borderline offensive impersonation that sounded nothing like the real Joe, based on a couple of phrases I've heard him use, once when he accidentally punched himself in the chin and said 'Silly sausage!' and another time, apropos of his hair, when he said, 'Look at my barnet!'

Later LADbible released video clips and went large on the 'Joe Wicks impression', to my shame, should he ever hear it.

There is talk of loosening the lockdown. Some DIY stores may reopen. But social distancing will apparently remain in place until December. This is the 'new normal'. This is the new reality.

Thursday 23 April

At 8 p.m. we were playing cricket in the back garden.

'I'll be wicky,' Arthur said.

Ray, mishearing, said, 'Arthur's Wookie.'

Jack, who enjoys Ray's mispronunciations, leapt on this. 'Yeah! You can be Wookie! Can I be on your teen?'

There was a noise of cheering and clapping.

'What's that?' Arthur said.

'People clapping the NHS,' I said.

'Cringe!' Jack said.

We went out front and I clapped and Arthur clapped. Our next-door neighbour was outside too, banging a pot with a wooden spoon, and there was a sound of cheers and clattering, but I stayed in the doorway and didn't venture up to the front gate. We've lived on our road a couple of years but I still don't know many people on the street. I said to her, 'I'm sort of curious to see who the other neighbours are.'

'I think they're more curious to see you,' she replied.

It was cringe, but also not cringe, and whether or not it made any difference to any front-line workers, it felt like we were marking something, an urge to connect and see each other in terrible times and make something positive from it, and also saying, this is different. For good or ill, these times are special.

Nancy made a fish dish, with cumin and smoked paprika.

'Paprika is just BTEC chilli,' Jack said.

Monday 27 April

The news is starting to talk about lockdown maybe being not exactly lifted but ameliorated a little. Meanwhile, Trump delivered a press conference a day or two ago in which he mentioned the possibility of injecting people with disinfectant to cure them of Covid. They have now announced there will be no more White House press briefings.

Friday night was a watershed because, for the first time, Ray put himself to bed. For years, the routine has involved a nightly ritual of lying next to him until he falls asleep, which can take half an hour or more and sometimes involves several false starts if he wakes and hears you creeping away. Nancy and I do it on alternate nights and increasingly it's felt like a punishment for our failure to make the effort to sleep-train him properly in his early years. On Friday I was following the usual formula and attempting to quietly make my escape having read him his stories and lain next to him, but he was restless, and I was growing impatient because we were planning to watch a horror film called *Hush* and it was already getting late. He kept waking, and then after one of my exits he got cross and slammed the door shut after me. I went downstairs and for a while there was stomping. Then it went quiet. Half an hour later I went up, and he was asleep in bed with toys all over the floor, which he'd evidently strewn there in a fit of anger before conking out. It felt almost like a miracle, and probably a one-off, but he did it again on Saturday night, this time with Nancy telling him he'd get a reward, and again on Sunday. It is hard to overstate what a difference this will make to our lives and I feel very proud of him, and maybe a little foolish for not being firmer earlier.

Tonight he said he was afraid of the gap between his mattress and the wall. He thinks a monster is going to 'grab him'. Nancy stuffed it with pillows, which seemed to do the trick.

At supper, with a lot of cajoling, I prevailed on Arthur and Jack to help cook. Jack grated cheese for omelettes. Arthur made avocado toast – I showed him how to squeeze the lime juice and sprinkle the chilli flakes. In the big scheme of things it felt like a small but significant victory, spreading the burden of kitchen duties, even though with all the managerial oversight it requires, being helped probably ends up taking more time than not being helped.

As Arthur tucked in, I said to him, 'Now, doesn't it taste better knowing you made it yourself?'

'Not really,' he said. 'Tastes slightly worse if I'm honest.'

May 2020

WE'RE NOT MUTED

Saturday 2 May

Nancy had set up a Zoom call with her mum, Liz, for 6 p.m.

'She feels like she isn't speaking to us.'

With everyone locked down at home, these video conferences are the closest we now get to socializing. There are various apps to do it with – Skype, FaceTime, Chime, Teams – but for some reason the market leader is Zoom. Zoom is now so well established that there is an ancillary phenomenon of 'Zoom-bombing', which is when trolls hijack your conference by posting child porn or racist imagery, proving, once again, that there is no advance in technology that doesn't also bring with it a fresh opportunity for cruelty.

What's far more annoying about Zooms, though, is how glitchy they are, with people talking over one another, cutting out, and freezing.

On this occasion, the kids were already engrossed in their various screens, and I was conscious they might rebel. 'Hmm,' I said to Nancy. 'Not sure that's a good idea.'

'Come on, guys!' she said. She was at the kitchen table, with her laptop, waiting for the Zoom to start.

'But she isn't even on the call yet.'

'She is about to be. Come on. It isn't a lot to ask.'

I was making a supper, a jailhouse version of a Jamie Oliver savoury pancake recipe that was intended to use up various vegetables that were on the turn: two wrinkly peppers, a two-day-old baked potato, an aubergine, some floppy coriander and a red onion.

Nancy's mum came on the call. 'HOW ARE YOU ALL?'

'Good,' the boys said with low energy and some glances at their phones.

There were muttered off-screen threats from Nancy. *'Fine. You don't have to talk to her. But you can go to your room and there'll be no PlayStation.'* Ray was slouched out of shot on the sofa, having problems with a game on the iPad. 'I need heeeeelp. What can I dooooo?'

'Get Arthur to help,' I said. 'Art, can you help Ray?'

'I don't want Arthur to help.'

Nancy's mum said: 'WHAT HAVE YOU BEEN DOING?'

I'm thinking: *They've been indoors for seven weeks watching TV and playing video games and going mental.*

Jack: 'Not much. Some schoolwork and been in the garden a little bit.'

Nancy to Arthur: *'Get off the iPad.'*

'I told him to be on it,' I say. 'He's helping Ray.'

Meanwhile, the peppers are griddling and the potatoes frying and I'm measuring out a mug full of flour which the recipe calls for, and then, to chop the red onion finely, I pull out a Japanese cleaver which I don't use very often.

'ARE YOU READING ANYTHING?' Liz asks the boys.

'It's not *working*!' Ray says.

'I'm trying,' Arthur says. 'Hold on.'

'You can go to another room,' Nancy says. 'Sorry, Mum, it's a bit hectic here at the moment.'

And that's when I look down and see a thin slice of my index finger has been cleanly removed, a section of nail and digital topsoil sliced off. I have a heightened feeling of *am-I-seeing-what-I'm-seeing?* and *oh shit*, and a flash of recollection of a Sylvia Plath poem about cutting off the tip of her thumb while chopping an onion, in which she compares it to an 'Indian' scalping a pilgrim.

I take down the medical box and begin looking for supplies, a large plaster preferably. There seems to be nothing in there. Blood is trickling onto the floor. I need something to staunch it. I feel panicky.

'Guys, does anyone know if we have any plasters?'

Jack notices first. 'Mum! We need plasters!'

Nancy looks up. 'Mum, we have to go, Louis's cut his finger.'

'Dad, you look pale,' Arthur says.

Blood is splatting down in big drops. From a box of Halloween dressing-up materials, specifically the fixings for an Egyptian mummy outfit, Nancy has sourced some bandages, which I secure in place with brown packing tape.

'Don't use that!' Nancy says. 'You need to run it under the tap first.'

'No, I think I need to staunch the bleeding.'

'You'll never get the tape off.'

'I will.'

'Why don't we have any *actual plasters*?' Jack says.

In the midst of all this I was having flashbacks to the sight of the finger and the slice, how much was gone, what it had looked like, and the fact that the blood, while it was trickling, was definitely not spurting. At the end of last year I'd done a Hostile Environments Course, in preparation for the possible story about radicalized UK jihadis in detention camps in Iraq and Syria, which involved spending a week in the Kent countryside learning what to do in the event of massive head trauma and loss of limbs. And here I was, now panicking and floundering after a tiny digital amputation. I couldn't remember what I was supposed to do. Maybe nothing? There was no question of going to hospital, amid the hordes of Covid patients. The only thing that came to mind was to raise my finger to reduce pressure. So I walked around with it up, like a kitchen jihadi pointing at the hereafter.

'Dad, you look pale,' Art said again.

Also, unlike some cuts, it actually was painful. One thing I didn't feel ready to do was carry on with the fucking Jamie Oliver pancakes.

'I'm going for a lie-down,' I said, and carrying my finger before me like a badly wounded but beloved small pet, I went upstairs and lay down.

A few minutes later, I came downstairs and ate the pancakes, which Nancy had put the finishing touches to, and took a couple of Nurofen. I went to bed, awaking at 3 a.m. to considerable pain. My finger was throbbing. Jesus Christ, it was *really throbbing*. I went downstairs and with some difficulty I peeled off the brown packing tape. The wound looked less bad than I feared. Blood dribbled out but it looked as though I'd just planed a narrow slice off my finger and nail. I ran it under the tap. This was more painful than I expected. I was sweating and I grew dizzy. I felt ridiculous. My head filled with absurd images of myself as a pirate in an old movie slurping grog and chomping down on a knife as the ship's surgeon amputated my leg. I wrapped a paper towel loosely around the finger then lay on a sofa. It started feeling better. The next day – today – I went to the chemist.

'I sliced a little bit off the end,' I said. 'Do you want to see it?'

'It looks like a deep cut,' she said. 'The risk is it gets infected. They used to do an iodine spray. But we have these non-adhesive iodine patches. You can cut off little strips. And we have dressings, but take them off at night.'

I went off with a spring in my step, feeling vindicated by the chemist. *A deep cut.* Hah! I wonder how long before it will feel normal again.

In other news, I called Marce. He said he'd attended a few Zoom-based drinks parties with our mutual friend Tom Hodgkinson, the *Idler* editor. 'It's awful,' he said. 'No one can hear you. It's like being Bruce Willis in *The Sixth Sense*.'

Monday 4 May

I posted on Instagram about my injury and Jamie Oliver reached out. He says Japanese knives can be more hazardous to use because they are angled 'just on one side' unlike European blades, which have a v-shaped edge. He described an incident when he was on TV in Japan, sliced his finger, but had to play it off and keep cooking because it was live – presumably feeding parts of his flesh and blood to the Japanese equivalent of Greg Wallace.

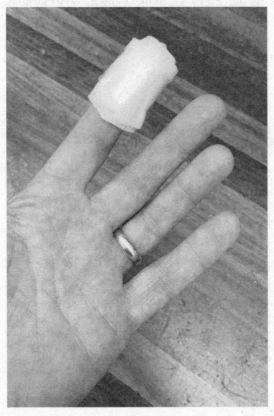

Digital carnage.

Tuesday 5 May

For the second day running, Joe Wicks's wife Rosie was doing his slot. For weeks he hasn't been able to use one of his hands, do squat thrusts, the plank, push-ups, etc., after hurting it falling off his bike. He was struggling on Friday. Monday, he got Rosie to fill in while he stood off to one side in a suit, calling out trivia questions. 'In what country would you find Machu Picchu? My mum went there.'

Nancy is starting to resent me doing it every morning.

Sunday 10 May

Listless today. It was the first time I've actually felt confused and forlorn and not quite known what to do with myself. Trying to keep kids off the phone, running around and saying, 'Want to play Quirkle?' No one did.

In the evening we did a Zoom quiz with Nancy's family; her mum and four brothers and in-laws. It's something we've started doing as a way of socializing online without everything descending into a free-for-all of crosstalk. Different households take it in turns to host. Tonight Nancy's mum, Liz, was quizmaster. At the beginning there's always some faffing. We'd just finished supper and I was clearing plates.

'Just sit next to me,' Nancy said. 'It looks like I'm on my own. *Hi Mum! Hi Ernesto!*'

'You're still muted,' Arthur said.

'No, we're not.'

The question of whether you're muted or unmuted turns out to be surprisingly fraught. You don't want to give away your answers by announcing them to everyone. You also don't want to spend time talking to a screen of people who can't hear anything you're saying.

Liz had included a literary round. 'HOW MANY WRITERS HAVE WON THE BOOKER PRIZE TWICE? BONUS POINT FOR THE NAMES OF THE WRITERS.'

'Definitely Hilary Mantel and Peter Carey,' I said. '*Liz, to qualify for the bonus points, do you have to get the number right? And how many names can you put down? Because in theory you could just put down a hundred names.*'

'*Dad!*' Arthur said. My question had annoyed him.

A little later he was grappling on top of Jack, who was on a yellow armchair.

'Get off him NOW!' Nancy said.

I checked to see if we were muted.

Arthur left and Jack looked ruffled and upset: 'You're the worst flipping parents in the universe.'

Round 2 was portraits of writers – my dream subject. I became super-focused, tuning out all family mayhem, and tried to take custody of the pencil.

'Let me write them down,' I said. 'I know these. Somerset Maugham. T. S. Eliot. Tennyson . . .'

The pencil was still not in my grasp so I made a lunge for it. 'I'll do it.'

'Why are you so grumpy?' Nancy said.

'We're running out of time.'

'Can you at least act like you're having a good time?' Nancy said.

'I am having a good time.'

'RIGHT, HERE ARE YOUR ANSWERS.'

In the end, we lost by half a point to family members in New Malden.

Nancy was disconsolate. I was aware we were both at risk of using passive-aggression to blame the other one for the loss.

'I knew there were twenty-seven books in the New Testament,' Nancy said. 'I don't know why I put twenty-six.'

'I'm more puzzled why you thought there are five strings on a cello.'

'Seriously, you're bringing that up?'

'I'm not making a big thing out of it.'

'Why are you bringing that up?'

'There are four strings on a violin and on a double bass. I wondered why you thought there were more on a cello. Maybe there are on a viola. I don't know. I'm not making a big thing out of it. I'm genuinely confused.'

The Zoom quiz clashed with an official announcement from

Boris about the status of the lockdown. The new message, which has replaced 'Stay At Home', is 'Stay Alert'. No one seems too clear on what it really means, or whether we are still in lockdown, and when, if ever, it will end. You are allowed to go to the park and meet one other person, if they are two metres away. A reporter at the press conference asked if that meant you were supposed to leave the park if there was more than one person you recognized. No clear answer was forthcoming.

Wednesday 13 May

Last night I did my podcast with Chris O'Dowd, who is in LA. It's the last of the series – number ten – but it was stressful for various reasons, not least because I worried I was presuming on our friendship to get him to do it. It had been late when I texted him about the arrangement, and I only half read his reply, failing to notice that he'd suggested a different day. The upshot being that on Monday, while putting down Ray, Nancy called me to say Chris was wondering where I was. I apologized and we did the call on Tuesday instead, and it went fine – he was great, witty and warm, as he always is – while I was conscious of being tired and babbling at various points – wanting to prise something intimate out of him but also not wanting to take the conversation into awkward terrain. I decided to open the conversation with a flattering preamble about the joy he brings to his audiences, then slid into a question about the celebrity rendition of 'Imagine' that amused the Internet so much at the beginning of lockdown.

'It was a Vera Lynn thing?' I said. 'Some commented that it was worse than the actual pandemic.'

'I think it was you that said that.'

Chris and his wife Dawn have a child Ray's age and another two years younger. It was reassuring to compare notes with a fellow parent of a young family struggling in ways that felt very familiar. The stresses are real. From him – or maybe from someone else – I heard it said: no one has tried to do this before, combine caring for small children at home with a full-time job. It is a mission you can't win. An exercise in total frustration for all parties.

In Coronaland, lockdown is loosening but it's confusing – exactly what's allowed and what isn't – and apparently there are mini-relapses wherever the rules are relaxed.

Friday 15 May

Today my director Tom came by, with a mask on his face, refusing all offers of tea or coffee. It was my first physical encounter with a work colleague, other than Nancy, since mid-March. It felt weirdly normal. Maybe that's not that surprising. What is it supposed to feel like? A reunion? A transport of ecstasy? It was just nice to have a different energy in the house – someone to play host to a bit and to cater to and chat and catch up with.

We were filming interstitial moments for our four-part look-back at my old programmes. Depressingly, it appears there is a mini-glut of these kinds of series which feature old material repackaged and linked with present-time interviews and Zoom calls to former interviewees. Romesh Ranganathan has done one. A Michael Palin one is in the works. The challenge is to draw out resonances, to make it more than the sum of its parts. Early on, I had been pushing for something a little arty-farty, maybe in an Adam Curtis vein, with the footage you would never normally see: out-takes of me talking to my directors and sound recordists miking up contributors and accidental shots of feet because we didn't realize the camera was on, accompanied by deep reflections on how reality is constructed in documentaries. 'Whether you are making fiction or documentary, the one tends inevitably towards the other,' Jean-Luc Godard once said, in a quote I can't seem to find on the Internet. Anyway, my pretentious vision has mercifully died and fallen by the wayside. In place of it, Arron came up with four simple themes: faith, commerce, law and order, and family, as a way of imposing a shape on clips from different shows made over twenty-five years.

In the upstairs bedroom, I'd dug out battered old boxes from the loft, with letters and documents and notebooks dating from my twenties and thirties. There were the journals I'd kept while trying to write my first book, *The Call of the Weird*, and I was struck by the hundreds of pages of unused material, and the sense of compulsive, almost pathological productivity that had gone into them, and how far the finished work had fallen from being what I'd hoped it would be. I thought about rewriting the book, which would almost certainly be a crazy thing to do. I found file after file filled with newspaper cuttings that I'd thought might make subjects for documentaries, about weird crimes and cults and fetishes. And articles I'd written, and one interview with me from the *TV Nation* zine, a fan-photocopied leaflet. 'Louis Theroux Speaks' was the headline. It had been the first time I'd ever been interviewed – I was excited, talking about the segment I'd done about the Ku Klux Klan. I'd hoped it would be the first of many interviews, though it would be several years before I was asked to do another one, and it was embarrassing to reflect on how intent I'd been on success and how excited and hopeful of becoming famous, all those years ago, brimming with ambition and racked with self-doubt.

I had the sensation of ascending a slope, and pausing to look back at the view, gazing out over the vista of the lived years for a moment, a small sensation of accomplishment that one feels a little ashamed of indulging, before pressing on towards the summit.

Tuesday 19 May

The day before my birthday.

Increasingly, I hear disgruntlement over the whole notion of the lockdown. The feeling that it was at best misguided, unscientific, and possibly something more sinister: an attempt to control. I also hear frustration at the public's willingness to go on with the lockdown plan, sheep-like and brainwashed. Along with Covid there is now a secondary pandemic of indignation. 'It's a scandal that . . .' – the sentence can go anywhere from there. That teachers aren't going back to work. That they *are* going back. That lockdown is ending. That it isn't ending. That so many old people are dying. That so many younger people are cooped-up and the economy is being banjaxed over questionable data about deaths and infection paths.

The only thing keeping me sane at the moment is Joe Wicks. That's silly. Of course other things are keeping me sane. Doing the podcasts. Cooking for the family. Cleaning and tidying. Mindhouse winning commissions – for my projects and also now for the Jeremy Bamber series and a possible three-parter to be presented by podcast host and DJ Alice Levine. But exercise is the foundation. If nothing else happens in the day, at least you know you've accomplished something if you've done some hard physical exercise.

Thursday 21 May

Yesterday was my birthday. I took a day off from my diary. The plan, prior to lockdown, had been to have a big party at a pub in Harlesden, which Nancy had been arranging. Not something I've done before – my birthdays are usually low-key affairs, with a few friends coming over. But the big five-oh had felt like it warranted something on a grander scale.

With pub option gone, kicked into the future, Nancy had arranged a compilation of happy birthday messages from friends and family. I watched it when I woke up, still cobwebbed with dreams, a parade of loving and friendly faces from different phases of my life. Some did skits, some sang or just spoke from the heart or regaled me with compliments, and there was a sense of everyone compensating for us being in lockdown, which made it more special: *here we are in these strange times doing our best*. Some of them, out of context and with lockdown hair, for a second or two I struggled to recognize.

Afterwards I felt both touched and also unworthy. I was trying to make some sense of it, and it may be that being deprived of outside human contact, I was going into overload. The truth was, I wasn't sure what I was feeling – certainly gratitude, also a sense of not deserving my friends, that they and especially Nancy had gone to a lot of trouble, and was I who they thought I was? I was struggling to recognize myself in their love.

I told her, 'Thanks so much, Nancy. I love it. I'm very lucky.' But mainly what made me happy was to see how much it meant to her, and her uncomplicated pleasure in doing something for me.

The day was a succession of Zoom calls with friends and family members. 'Maybe we'll do the big party at the pub next year,' Nancy said.

Among the many gifts that came in: a bread recipe book, some espadrilles, two bottles of posh tequila, a wooden cookbook holder, a David Bowie poster, and a karaoke machine. In the evening we cranked it up and Ray sang 'Greased Lightnin'' like someone in a trance, mesmerized by the screen. 'Go greased lightning you're burning up the corner of my eye.'

I sang 'Every Day Is Like Sunday' which seemed all-too-appropriate in Covidland. Then with Nancy I sang 'Under Pressure'.

'People on the streets. Ba-da-dee-dah-dah.'

Afterwards, we went to bed and cuddled.

'Did you enjoy it?'

'I loved it. Thanks, Nancy. I'm so lucky to have you.'

Sunday 24 May

Ritual Zoom quiz with Nancy's family. The East Finchley contingent set the questions and the scoring system was erratic. Half points, double points. There was no logic. The rounds we were strong in seemed cruelly points-poor. Still, we were holding on to our lead until the end, when a picture round about sport did for us.

After the quiz, we all caught up for a few minutes. Nancy vented about the lockdown, which she viewed as too strict, and the over-cautious approach to school return. Until a few days ago it seemed Ray would be back at school from 1 June. But that now looks unlikely. Nancy feels the teachers' unions aren't giving enough consideration to children's well-being. It is possible the kids will be out of school until September.

Nancy's brother John pushed back gently. Ernesto, another brother, who lives on his own, was saying: 'I have had enough of this country. I want to leave. This is it for me. People don't understand what it's like living on your own. The loneliness. And I'm better off than most because I have work to go to.'

Milton, another of Nancy's four brothers, said, 'But where are you going to go? There are lockdowns everywhere.'

Earlier in the day, while mowing the lawn, I had listened to an episode of the Joe Rogan podcast from a couple of weeks ago. He was interviewing the engineer and rocketeer Elon Musk. With his plans for tunnels under Los Angeles and space probes and colonies on Mars, Musk came across like a character in a Marvel movie, a combination of Tony Stark and Doc Ock. He was championing some kind of brain implant – it seemed he wanted to turn people into cyborgs. In fact, he said, we're *already* cyborgs. Glasses, pros-thetics, even phones are all mechanical enhancements that make us part machine. He has just had a baby and given her a name that is unpronounceable, employing an orthography that is without any discernible legibility. He spoke very slowly and without any apparent attempt to amuse, which gave him a surprising oracular power. The pauses, the breaths for thought – I found myself hanging on the words.

Both Musk and Rogan are Covid sceptics. Musk said the data is unreliable. Too many cases are being chalked up to coronavirus, when the infected person may have died from being knocked over by a bus. Hospitals are not crowded, contrary to popular belief, they said. I don't know whether this is true or what to think. They say the pandemic may serve as a helpful dry run for a real pandemic in the future.

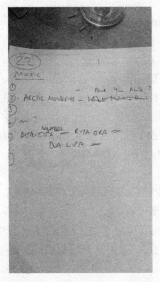

Seriously struggling on the music round.

Thursday 28 May

I was doing Joe Wicks. Nancy said, 'Are you going to hoover the carpet afterwards?'

'RIGHT, THIRTY-FIVE SECONDS OF SILLY BILLIES! COME ON!'

Me out of breath. 'Yes, OK.'

'You know I'd love to be doing Joe Wicks, but there are a million things that need doing.'

'OK.'

'I just feel bad for Ray.'

'He's fine.'

'He's spending so long on screens . . .'

'TEN MORE SECONDS! KEEP IT GOING! I LOVE THIS SONG. GEORGE EZRA!'

'Nancy, PLEASE! This is the one thing in the day that I actually NEED to do. Don't make it about Joe Wicks.'

'I just think it's selfish.'

'OK, MEGASPIN! LET'S SEE WHAT THE WHEEL SAYS. OH NO. FROG JUMPS AGAIN!'

'You're sweating on the carpet.'

'TINY SPIN! LET'S SEE WHAT HAPPENS. WHAT? MOUN-TAIN CLIMBERS. THERE'S SOMETHING WRONG WITH THE WHEEL. IT'S NOT LEVEL. RIGHT, THIRTY-FIVE SECONDS OF MOUNTAIN CLIMBERS.'

Friday 29 May

Awoke with a hangover having drunk more than usual due to anxiety brought on by two cuts I'd watched of the archive shows, neither of which was showing signs of working. *Stay up*, I thought. *This music sounds good, maybe another drink, even though it's 11.30.*

Today I did Joe Wicks with Nancy and Jack while Ray watched YouTube. It was Fancy Dress Friday and Joe was wearing a panda head and doing push-ups. I admired his dedication to the cause, wearing an outfit that would be liable to suffocate you even if you weren't doing a high-intensity cardio workout. I sometimes wonder how many children are actually doing the sessions – based on the data set of my own household, the under eighteens are at best only intermittent participants. Does he need to wear the panda head? But mainly I was happy that on this occasion I *wasn't* doing it alone and that I was being joined by my wife and child, keeping the blues at bay with vigorous physical exercise.

In the evening, Nancy was on Ray duty. Outside his bedroom I eavesdropped on her reading him a new story, *Monsters Don't Eat Princesses*. He was rapt, staring at the drawings, as they both lay under the covers. He looked younger than I expected. *He's still only five*, I thought. Still not much more than a toddler. Still living between the real world and a magical world of his imagining. I went downstairs and got my phone and came up and recorded a little bit. Just caught the end of Nancy reading and Ray leaning over and picking up a vuvuzela, a souvenir brought back by friends who were at the South Africa World Cup in 2010, and blowing softly into it.

In other news, my finger – the one I sliced weeks ago – is almost completely better. But I do think there is a little bit missing.

June 2020

BUBBLES

Tuesday 2 June

Last night I had my first alcohol-free night in about three or four months – possibly more – just to see what it felt like. Main observation was a steep dip in the pleasure centres of my brain, increased boredom, plus mild sense of smugness. Weirdly, not much noticeable difference to grogginess levels the following morning.

The other side effect was heightened alertness, leading to the ability to dominate without mercy in three consecutive games of Confident, the quiz game, with Arthur, Nancy and Nancy's brother Ernesto, who joined us remotely from his place in the West Country. Jack got annoyed mid-game and left. After a few minutes, he called out: 'Arthur!' Arthur went over to the TV room. 'He's changed my Netflix profile name to Flare-Nostrils and my picture to a pair of slugs.'

It was Ernesto's birthday. He was turning forty-eight.

'It's a great number,' he said. 'Forty-seven was prime. Forty-eight has so many factors. Two, four, six. Is three one?'

'I don't know,' I said. 'Twelve is. So three must be.'

Ernesto, who works in one of the caring professions, is doubtful of authority and received wisdom. Possibly a Covid denier of some kind.

'I'm not a Covid denier,' he said.

'A Covid sceptic.'

'Nah.'

'A Covid refusenik?' I said.

'Nah. I'm a *Covid renegade*.'

Nancy, upset with schools still not being back, and uncharacteristically at odds with the unions, is also a Covid-something – maybe *maverick*? She has access to alternative news sources via her Twitter account and she's been posting non-mainstream lockdown-sceptical content online. 'I've alienated a lot of my Labour Party colleagues,' she said. 'One said, "Fine, when children start dying I'll be sure to send you a picture of the corpses."'

In the US there is unrest following a viral clip showing police in Minneapolis killing a black man called George Floyd, after he'd been arrested for supposedly using a fake $20 bill. One of the officers, Derek Chauvin, knelt on Floyd's neck for more than nine minutes, despite Floyd being handcuffed and repeatedly saying he couldn't breathe. Floyd was forty-six years old and had been working as a bouncer in a nightclub, which had closed due to Covid. A random fact, passed along by my director Tom, who like me is a fan of rap, is that George Floyd had performed on two DJ Screw albums under the moniker Big Floyd.

One or two rappers and community activists I've met in Milwaukee and Mississippi have been organizing protests, while Nick Fuentes, from our postponed film about the far right, has been livestreaming himself taking to the streets in a lavender Hawaiian shirt trolling the protesters. 'We're supporting the cause! We're down with Soros!' he says. Then, spying an interracial couple: 'Looks like we have some race mixing.' For many on the far right, the upheaval is a delight, affirming their view that racial conflict is inevitable.

Wednesday 3 June

Nancy was awake at 7.15.

I said, 'What time is it?'

'Seven fifteen. I've been awake since five.'

'Go back to sleep!'

'I can't sleep. I've been waking up at five the last three mornings. I'm feeling so upset.' She was crying.

'Go back to sleep.'

'I can't sleep.'

'You need to get more exercise,' I said.

'I can't believe you just said that.'

She left the room and went downstairs. I got up and made her a cup of tea.

'I'm sorry, Nancy.'

She was under a blanket on the sofa, apparently trying to get back to sleep. I unloaded the dishwasher and tidied the kitchen.

'I'm going down to the Co-op,' I said. 'We're out of dishwasher tablets.' Then, remembering myself, I asked, 'Do you want to talk?'

'No.'

I had woken up feeling possibly less groggy and more healthy than normal after a second night without alcohol. After a Joe Wicks, I checked what Ray was watching on YouTube. At his request, I searched up a show that was supposed to feature a small boy gaming, but instead there was a girl.

'This isn't RonaldOMG,' I said.

'It's GamerGirl and RonaldOMG,' he said. Then, with the air of someone who's figured something out, he said, 'Dad, what is the opposite of Netflix?'

'Tell me.'

'Amazon.'

'OK,' I said, thinking the answer made a kind of sense, and wondering: What *is* the opposite of Netflix? Maybe a Neanderthal scribbling on a cave wall? Or maybe someone running through a field of wild flowers? Or simply the absence of Netflix?

We had arranged a work call for 11 a.m. Then I remembered my mum and her husband, Michael, were coming over, our first visit since the beginning of lockdown. They arrived around 10.30, came up the side passage and sat on the wooden deck in the garden.

'How's your health?' I asked Michael. 'Have you recovered from the Covid?'

I'd been told by my mum that Michael had been through several phantom cases of the virus, self-isolating and following all the protocols, before coming out and acknowledging he may, on this occasion, have been mistaken.

'It turned out to be a false alarm,' Michael said. 'But thank you for your concern.'

'Michael's had it two or three times now,' my mum said. 'It's a miracle he's still alive.'

I offered them coffee. They seemed in two minds about accepting it.

'We haven't really been observing lockdown,' I said. I'm not sure why I said it, since we have. Then I heard myself ranting about schools being closed.

'Did you see the issue of the *New York Times* where they turned the whole front page into a memorial honouring the dead?' I asked. 'They were mostly in their nineties. I hadn't realized it skewed *that* old. Do you know the average age of death from Covid? It's higher than the average life expectancy. It's like eighty-something.'

Even as I was saying this, I was aware it was crass, given that Michael is in fact over eighty, but I ploughed on.

'It just feels like there's something they're not telling us. It's like the whole masks thing. First they were telling us not to wear them, because they don't work, and in the next breath they were telling us they needed them for staff in hospitals. It's like they think we're children and we won't notice.'

'You're preaching to the converted,' my mum said. 'I've been enjoying your podcasts. I wasn't sure about the one with the actress.'

'Rose McGowan.'

'Yes, there was something about her.'

It had been a feisty interview, with a talented actor and survivor of sexual abuse, who'd called out the predatory movie producer Harvey Weinstein and his alleged Hollywood enablers.

'I think I know what you mean,' I said. 'It seems to have divided people. I just enjoyed the conflict of it. I don't like it when they get too cosy.'

'Well, you see, I like cosy,' Mum said. 'Lenny Henry. Now that was a good one.'

'I don't like cosy,' I said. 'I like fractious.'

I asked if they knew anyone who'd died from Covid, and my mum mentioned an old friend, a feminist writer and critic of some distinction. Towards the end she'd lived in a care home not far from our house. 'But she hadn't been well for some time,' Mum said. 'She'd had dementia and the last couple of times I saw her she hadn't recognized me. It was rather upsetting.'

'How do you mean?'

'Well, the last time I saw her she didn't recognize me and she got cross with me and Michael had to smooth it over. And the time before that, she'd had all these soft toys and teddy bears on her shelves and she'd just look at them and say, "Isn't that *interesting*?" Over and over again.'

'Well, it's like this phrase they keep saying on the radio. "Every death is a tragedy." If you lead a full and wonderful life and then you get dementia, aged a hundred and five, and then you die from Covid, it's sad, but is it in fact a *tragedy*? People act as though it's not natural to die.'

'They used to call pneumonia the old man's friend,' Michael said. When they left, we bumped arms.

'I've been hugging some people,' I said.

'Have you?'

'But I suppose you can't be too careful.'

Afterwards I felt a dump of guilt and shame, an acrid release of self-reproach, sensing I'd been less than friendly or less friendly than I might have been, begrudging somehow, with everything going on and after so long without seeing them. I realized a nasty side of me was – in a completely unfair way – resentful of them. I envied their lack of responsibilities. Some dark part of me was annoyed at them for what we were going through. I envied the calm I imagined infused their lives. And at the same time I battled the resentment I was feeling, and I had a vision of myself as an Eskimo shoving his ageing parent onto an ice floe and pushing her out to sea.

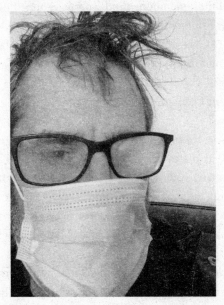

Loving the new normal.

Friday 5 June

George Floyd protests everywhere.

I got up with Ray at around seven. The previous night we had been at our regular local pub quiz, via Zoom, hosted by two local dads. A virtual gallery of middle-class front rooms and kitchens. The tableau and the unexpected intimacy of being a virtual guest in so many homes at once was strangely comforting. I had a vision of ourselves as survivors of an apocalypse, all of us in bunkers around the city, a remnant joining together and forming a kind of underground – though, granted, not to mount any kind of resistance but simply to answer questions on countries that begin with K and pictures of celebrities as children. We were joined remotely by local friends who were on separate screens – in an arrangement that involved multiple phones and laptops propped up around the kitchen table, some of them needing to be muted.

At the start I was upstairs, delayed by filming. Nancy texted.

What is the longest river in Italy? she asked.

The Tiber?

What about France?

The Rhône?

Both of these answers were wrong. When I came down we drank Prosecco and as the evening wore on we drifted into an argument about performative outrage on the Internet. The spectacle of bland celebrities and influencers with no track record of working for social justice putting up black squares on their Instagram feeds, supposedly in solidarity with Black Lives Matter. Nancy was having none of it.

'They all vote Tory and send their children to private schools and then cry about police brutality,' she said. 'The only person that promised anything like real systemic change they pilloried.'

The topic moved on to Barack Obama and whether he'd changed anything.

'He imprisoned Chelsea Manning and *put her in isolation*,' Nancy said. 'It's basically torture!'

'Well, didn't he also pardon Chelsea Manning?' I said. 'Doesn't that count for anything?'

'Right after he tortured her!'

I was sailing into choppy water but too drunk to resist. I said: 'Well, you're making the best the enemy of the good.' And then knowing it would irritate her and enjoying the sonority of a trite phrase, I said: 'Politics is the art of the possible.'

'I'm sorry, but come on. He did nothing. What did he do? He did absolutely nothing! The kill list? The drone strikes?'

'Nancy prefers Trump to Clinton,' I said.

'*Ha ha*,' Nancy said.

'Hand on heart, do you see any difference between them?'

'Oh, come on. "*No there's no difference.*" Of course, there's a *difference*. Though in fact, since he's basically an isolationist and doesn't invade anywhere, Trump probably has been better on foreign policy.'

When it was time for Ray to go up I read him *The Cat in the Hat Comes Back*. He chose it. I was drunk by then and found it brilliant, with tiny cats emerging from a succession of hats, one for each letter of the alphabet, and under the last hat a magical energy called 'Voom'!

Then I came downstairs and drank a new brand of bourbon I'd found called Tin Cup, mixing it with grapefruit juice, and sat in the dark feeling sozzled and soppy, like the old man at the end of the bar, looking for answers in the bottom of his glass.

In bed, Nancy said an email had come in on the company website from someone who had been in touch with Joe Exotic. It said Joe was trying to get a message out to me from prison.

Saturday 6 June

Jack: 'What are we doing today?'

Nancy: 'We're going to a weirdo park.'

It was cold and rainy but we needed to get out, and so we drove to Regent's Park, bringing the Aerobie and some ginger loaf that was in the freezer, dense with molasses. Jack had made it weeks earlier from a Mary Berry recipe and it had been so heavy and gingery and so big – a slab, there was no other word for it – that it had gone uneaten. The ducks, geese and pigeons loved it though. The kids enjoyed pretending to be chased by the birds as they carried big hunks of the ginger loaf in their hands, screaming and running away and imagining they were about to be devoured by the geese and swans. At a socially distanced and largely empty park cafe we bought takeaway pizza, and a falafel wrap for Jack. It started to rain and we ate the food under a tree. When the rain stopped we walked through the rose gardens, where the roses were in full bloom. I went through the colours with Ray.

'I can see some purple ones. And orange. And pink,' he said.

I encouraged him to press his nose up close to one, 'Can you smell it?'

'Stop waffling, Dad. It literally doesn't smell of anything,' Jack said.

'It does, Jack! Bend in.'

'They don't smell of anything! Cringe. *Oooh I love the smell of roses.*'

But then, after sniffing the flowers in bed after bed, he agreed that some did smell a bit. We passed more beds and I looked back, after ten minutes or so, to see the two older boys with their faces in the blooms, inhaling.

Tuesday 9 June

Tom came over, we filmed and watched cuts, and then at four I stopped and took Ray to the local park. As an incentive, to get him off his iPad, I'd told him we could bring his Imaginext play figures, and when we arrived we positioned them on a couple of rocks in the playground, having hopped the fence and ignored the ragged caution tape. Kids kept wandering up to gawp at the figures.

'Sorry, I wish I could let you play with them, but there's a virus going round,' I said, feeling like a tit.

'Wow, so many Batmans,' said one of them, a six-year-old called Ollie. 'Why do you have so many?'

'We bought different packs and he came in more than one pack. Two metres. Sorry.'

'I know. I'm back at school now.'

He wandered off and for a while played with a friend, an older girl, presumably a sister, who was acting as chaperone. Then, unable to resist, he ran over and flicked one of Ray's figures with his finger, in violation of all Covid protocols. I gave the sister a hard stare.

'Come on, Dad,' Ray said, wanting me to take a more active role in the play-figure scenario.

Rousing myself, I began, 'So, Harley Quinn said, *"What are you doing here?"* And Batman said, *"Are you ready to battle?"'*

'Come on, Dad.'

'Come on what? I'm telling you what happened. Then Reverse Flash said, *"You think you can defeat me?"'*

I was flagging. The kid wandered back again.

'Hi Ollie,' I said. 'Sorry, I wish you could play with them. When this is over you can, I promise.'

He backed off to the fence, five or six metres away, and said, with chastening sarcasm, 'Is this far enough?'

Saturday 13 June

Total Covid deaths in the UK as of today: 41,662. Families are now allowed to socialize with one other family in a bubble. Bubble is the new word. Articles in the papers saying Boris Johnson should reduce the social distancing rule to one metre instead of two. The economy has shrunk 20 per cent, the biggest slide since records began. Nancy said yesterday that there is going to be a second spike – October through Feb, I think. I don't know where she heard it.

More George Floyd protests – it feels as though we are in the midst of a convulsive moment of moral reckoning brought on – in part – in reaction to lockdown. On 5 June my dad sent me an email mentioning a book he'd read at university, *The True Believer* by Eric Hoffer. He'd recalled a line, which he'd recently looked up, stating that the most perfect conditions for mass social upheaval, far more than a political crisis or economic distress, is that the populace should be completely bored.

I looked up Eric Hoffer. I'd imagined he might be bookish, an academic, a lecturer at Harvard, but in fact he was a more multi-faceted and mysterious character: the son of German immigrants, born in the Bronx, he'd been a migrant worker and a longshoreman – a docker – and had continued his manual labour even into his later life, long after he'd achieved literary success in the field of 'social psychology'.

Ongoing debates about whether it's OK for statues to come down. Some random civilian was in the news for having appointed himself protector of a statue of Boy Scouts founder Lord Baden-Powell. Specific grounds for the proposed cancellation of Baden-Powell unclear – his stand as a colonialist? His staunch opposition to masturbation? Today reports of Britain First – a far-right group – staging demonstrations around the West End, surrounding the

Churchill statue (which is inside a protective box), singing 'He's one of our own.' Some apparently wearing military helmets. Leader Paul Golding in a 'White Lives Matter' T-shirt. The Football Lads Alliance were also there. They attacked police, which seems off-brand, for a pro-Churchill authoritarian movement.

For the last two weeks it's felt as though we were in a new phase of the pandemic. Maybe the semi-loosened lockdown phase? The we-can-sort-of-see-people-illicitly phase. The lockdown has lost a bit of its glamour and excitement. It's more boring and maybe more annoying? There are no shortages, there are no special news conferences, there is less of a sense of doom. Just a dreariness and an atmosphere of anger and futility, and increasingly a generalized resentment that is finding expression in mass movements.

At supper the subject of Black Lives Matter came up.

'ACAB means All Cops Are Bastards,' Arthur said. 'But it doesn't mean literally all police. Just like "Fuck Tha Police" isn't about all police.'

'Language, Art,' I said.

'You're not making any sense,' Jack said. 'All cops *means* all police.'

Earlier they had been debating the ethics of throwing a statue of a slave trader into Bristol Harbour.

'They shouldn't have a statue of a slave trader,' Art said.

'Still,' Jack said, 'that's private property. You can't just go around destroying stuff.'

'He was literally a murderer,' Arthur said.

Changing the subject, Jack said, 'Do you know on the dark web you can order human leather, like a purse or something?'

Arthur said, 'Apparently if you search "wardrobe" on eBay and filter it by most expensive some of them are thirty grand because there's actually a person inside it. It's human trafficking.'

Then Jack said, 'I saw this thing today. Neil Armstrong was asked to swear on a Bible that he'd walked on the Moon and he refused to do it. There's a video of it.'

Arthur commented that Jeff Bezos was about to become the world's first trillionaire. 'If he wanted to, he could end climate change.'

'I'm not sure that's how it works,' I said.

'It would cost 300 billion to end climate change,' Arthur said.

Jack was sceptical. 'Who says?'

'It said so on *Bloomberg News*,' Arthur replied.

'Arthur's waffling so hard, he thinks he's some mad scientist.'

Sunday 14 June

It was the family Zoom quiz, hosted by the New Malden contingent. We opened up a big lead on the music round, identifying songs by random lyrics.

'MICHIGAN SEEMS LIKE A DREAM TO ME NOW.'

'Simon and Garfunkel. "America".'

'Are you sure?'

'*Yes*.'

'America. Not "Looking for America"?'

'Yes. I think so. But now you've got me questioning myself.'

'HE COULD PREACH THE BIBLE LIKE A PREACHER FULL OF ECSTASY AND FIRE.'

'*Wait, can you say that again? We didn't hear you?*'

'Ra Ra Rasputin.'

'*We're not muted*.'

Tuesday 16 June

A team meeting in the office. I cycled in. The tyres on my bike were soft and I couldn't find the keys for my bike lock. It was all so unfamiliar. It was the first time we've been in since March. There was a one-way system in effect in the building, entering through a side door I've never used before, and then out through the normal one. Me, Arron and Sophie crept around the abandoned office, where nothing had been touched for months – it was like a sunken ship or a house abandoned in a hurry after a volcanic eruption.

'No chance of a coffee, I suppose,' I said.

'The cafe's open but he needs thirty covers to make his numbers add up,' Sophie said.

Walking into Coterie, I saw the sad-faced manager and his new helper were wearing full facial covers – shiny welders' face masks. But there weren't many people around. I worried how he was going to make his thirty covers, and I thought about the effort they must have put in to make it Covid-safe and lay in the fresh supply of Danishes and cellophane-wrapped sandwiches. By lunchtime the cafe was closed. Had they thrown in the towel? Had they folded, gone home, tossed their tear-stained face masks in the bin?

At school pick-up I collected Ray and rode him back on the bike. He sat side-saddle then slipped off. He rode on the crossbar, then said, 'My willy's hurting.' I've had too many bikes stolen and never replaced the child seat, plus he's probably too heavy for most of them at this point. In the end he sprawled on the crossbar and I pushed the bike along with a foot on one pedal, like it was a scooter.

At home I put him on the iPad and made teas for me and Nancy and went upstairs.

'I've got a VO call about the podcast at four,' I said. 'That'll take forty-five minutes. Then I've got to send off the finalized speech for the corporate. Then I've got a Skype call at six.'

'Wait, what?'

'It's what's happening.'

'No, it isn't. I've got work too you know.' On her screen I saw 'Synanon'.

'Well, I'm sure we can make it work,' I said.

'I'm not making supper for the kids.'

'They can sort something out for themselves.'

'I am sick of you springing this shit on me,' she said. 'You didn't think to tell me in advance what was happening?'

'You're cc'd on all the emails!' This was a bluff. 'Forget the Synanon thing anyway. That's a lame-o idea!'

As I left the room she shouted after me: 'THAT'S NOT THE POINT, LOUIS. I'M SICK OF YOU PUTTING YOURSELF FIRST.'

I was tired and semi-manic. I shouted back: 'IT IS WHAT IT IS!'

Upstairs, the argument continued as I commenced a Zoom call.

'You always have it your way.'

'I don't have it my way! JESUS FUCKING CHRIST!'

This eruption of emotion came unexpectedly and from nowhere. I noticed the Velux windows were open and wondered how audible I was.

Wednesday 17 June

There were reports on the radio this morning about the price being paid by children for lockdown. Is it too high? They are voiceless and going through a mental health crisis. Over 1,500 paediatricians signed a letter to Boris Johnson saying that children's mental health needs are being jeopardized. A man from the teachers' union said: 'Schools have been open.'

'Bullshit,' Nancy said. 'Six schools. For key workers. Please.'

Yesterday we were talking about 'quality of life years'.

'I'm not trying to be weird,' I said, 'but someone aged a hundred in a bed with his tongue out living two extra years is not the same as a child's life being ended because of depression.'

'Exactly,' Nancy said.

In the evening I did a corporate event for a mysterious tech company via Zoom from the upstairs room. After my speech, I had remote drinks with the audience – they'd sent me mail-order cocktails. When I was finished, over supper, I had a couple more. Then with Nancy, I watched a true crime documentary series on Channel 4 called *Death in the Outback*.

Nancy went up. I tidied the kitchen, half-drunk, then sat at the kitchen table to write my diary when a text came in with a noise that sounded like *Zoop!* It said, **We have zero connection anymore.**

I just finished tidying the kitchen, I replied. **You're welcome.**

Then, feeling the stiff wind of indignation ballooning my sails, I wrote, **But I hope you've been having fun on Twitter. Or Instagram or whatever.**

Zoop! **That's not the point**, she wrote. **I'm upset at you treating me the same way you treat the kids. Trivialize.**

Zoop! Another text: **You take the piss out of me, and don't talk** to me in a normal way, you prod and tease, then you get angry. You're all over the place.

Zoop! And now you're drunk.

Fair enough. I was.

July 2020

LIFE ON THE EDGE

Wednesday 1 July

Interviewed on a new podcast by – guess who? – none other than Mr Spider-Man Lunges himself, Joe Wicks. His producer invited me on a few weeks ago and I didn't feel I could say no, given how much I've relied on his workouts during lockdown. I was delighted to learn he has watched and enjoyed many of my documentaries.

One of the strange features of doing the live sessions, after I'd gone public as a Wicks devotee in interviews in April, was that on more than one occasion, in the middle of workouts, he made remarks on-air that were directed *at me*. 'Come on, Louis Theroux! Let's see you doing the silly billies! Last ten seconds!' I can only compare it to what people in psychosis must experience when they imagine the TV is speaking to them. Exciting, yes, but also disconcerting.

Anyway, it was an honour to be on Joe's podcast and speak to him, via Zoom.

Naturally, I apologized for doing my very weird camp imper- sonation of him at the beginning of lockdown.

'It sounded nothing like you, Joe, and I don't know where it came from, and I'm sorry.'

He was very understanding.

He asked about times I've been filming and been afraid, and about Joe Exotic, of course. The premise of his podcast is to spread the word about wellness and health. Guests are invited to share a favourite tip of theirs. I mentioned that I'm a big believer in short naps, especially after lunch. This is something I've come to value more as I've grown older. Nancy thinks I may be narcoleptic, since the naps are on occasion involuntary. Naturally you can feel self- conscious napping at work – putting your head down on your desk and catching Zs in full view of the team. What I have tended to do instead is retire to a toilet cubicle for ten minutes or so, and sleep seated on the throne, head tilted forward.

I couldn't tell whether I sounded weird when I was talking about it.

Thursday 2 July

Nancy had a socially distanced book group at a friend's house. I put Ray down.

'Dad, you have to always breathe, otherwise you'll die, right?'

'Right.' Then I said: 'What if you forget to breathe?'

'Yeah. Or if you say a really long word.'

'Good point,' I said.

'Like badabadabadabadaanananananningningningnooooooohh,' he said.

'I guess you just have to be careful.'

'Dad, what is it when you crack the system?'

'What do you mean?'

'On *The Incredibles* they crack the system.'

'It's like solving a puzzle. You figure out the solution.'

'I thought it was like they broke it.'

'Well, they didn't break it, they figured it out.'

We read a book about being chased by a bear.

'Goodnight, Ray.'

'Dad, I don't want to go to school.'

'Oh, why not?'

'I don't want to grow up.'

'Well, it's not until Monday. So that's still four days away.'

'Dad. I don't want to be six. I want to be five. Or four.'

'You've got plenty of time to not grow up. Look at Arthur and Jack. They're much older and they're still young. Right, time to sleep.'

I tucked him in, thinking about him not wanting to grow up, hoping that it meant he was happy as he was and wanted to pause his life, and enjoy the simple pleasures of a five-year-old forever.

Friday 3 July

Did an old Joe Wicks from Dubai, downstairs in the front room while Ray was on the iPad.

Tom, my director, arrived at 10 a.m. or so and we filmed more off-the-cuff moments of me reflecting on old shows and finding things in boxes. You'd think it would be easier than doing straight voice-over but I end up having to do many retakes, and then out of frustration writing it, then trying to make it sound unrehearsed, which is almost impossible.

The radio is saying lockdown is loosening. Non-essential shops are already back, with social distancing. As of tomorrow, pubs open. Also hair salons. Maybe certain restaurants? I had a trepidatious feeling of 'this is life going back to normal' mixed in with a feeling of 'if it's normal, why does it feel so weird?' I think we are realizing that it may not be the same again for many months and even years. It won't blow over like a hurricane or a terrorist atrocity.

You can fly to certain countries for holidays now. They are graded by colour. According to risk. Like traffic lights. France, Germany, Iceland: OK. Portugal not OK. Greece, not for now but might be OK in a week or two. The phrase is 'air bridge'. America and Brazil definitely *not OK*. Boris Johnson was on the radio attempting to project calm. Worldwide deaths over half a million. Donald Trump in a death spiral, surely?

The local dads who host a Zoom pub quiz have decided to carry on. For some time we've felt confused, maybe a little peeved, at our consistently low showing in the standings, our failure to 'medal' or even reach anywhere near the podium. Tonight, purely as an experiment, to test our theory that other teams are using questionable methods, we cheated. It wasn't real cheating since we didn't enter our scores. But the weird thing was, we didn't even get within sight of the winners. Is something fishy going on? Or are we just not as clever as we think?

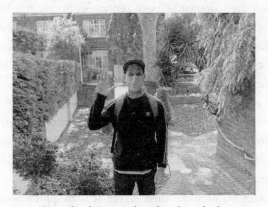

Tom the director, gloved and masked.

Tuesday 7 July

I headed into the office for a farewell workday. We have decided to give up the space we've been renting in Shepherd's Bush since it's not being used and there is no sign of change on the horizon. I cycled, navigating a route down through Queen's Park, Kensal Rise, Ladbroke Grove and North Kensington. I locked up my bike using a pair of chain locks, then went inside. The cafe, Coterie, has a new Perspex protective screen from counter to ceiling. The manager was making coffee but finished late morning again. Does he just give up out of despair halfway through the day or is his business plan to just make coffee for an hour or two and use pastries for display purposes only?

For lunch, we went out through the W12 shopping centre, Shepherd's Bush's apocalyptic mall, shops largely open, including the charity shop and socially distanced shoppers queuing outside Aldi, 30 per cent of people probably wearing masks. Across the Shepherd's Bush roundabout, the falafel van was closed, likewise Leon. Pret was open, though with depleted-looking stock.

We had meetings about story ideas. One about Derek Hay, a porn agent in Las Vegas who has been accused of operating an illegal prostitution scheme; another looking at misogynistic memes on the Internet called 'We Need to Talk About Karen' – mainly I just like the title, though the whole phenomenon of 'Karens' I find interesting: its sudden emergence as a cultural type, the square white woman in her thirties or forties who is perennially entitled and 'wants to speak to the manager', and the question of whether its use represents a calling out of power or is really just repackaged misogyny. The Joe Exotic idea is also inching forward – a few messages have gone back and forth between us via an intermediary in America. He wants to tell 'the real story', whatever that may mean.

And an idea for a series about snooker in the eighties – the heyday of Alex Higgins, Steve Davis and Jimmy White – which we are calling 'Ball Gods'. That one sprang out of a conversation about what we could make in lockdown, based mainly on archive footage and interviews that could be shot in a Covid-safe way.

At three thirty or so I knocked off and went outside to find my bike had gone. The chain was there, sliced through and left behind, like a serial killer's signature. My fourth bike stolen in ten months. I blamed myself for not using a D-lock and told myself it was a species of trickle-down economics – maybe whoever stole the bike really needed it – but I didn't really persuade myself, the job looked too efficient, and I had a vision of a syndicate sending out men with huge metal clippers in vans around London. *Lesson learned*, I thought. *For the fifth or tenth or hundredth time. Lesson fucking learned.*

I couldn't just hail an Uber – no mask – so I went over to the Overground. The main entrance was now exit only. Would I be allowed without a mask? I wasn't sure. I was relieved to see unmasked people on the platform.

Back at the house I only had fifteen minutes for an old Joe Wicks in which a fire alarm went off halfway through – the session was twenty seconds on, ten off, and was called something weird and Japanese-sounding like a *tatami* or *totato*. I made avocado toast and beans and reheated quiche for supper. Jack was complaining about lack of grapes so I took him off to the Co-op in Queen's Park and we bought grapes and strawberries. When I got back I ran a bath for Ray who was playing PlayStation with Nancy.

'Torture me, Dad.'

I tickled him, realizing, from the way I was overdoing the game, that I was tetchy and over-tweaked.

'I'm going to eat you, skinny bones,' I growled.

He giggled.

'I'm going to destroy you . . . until you die.'

'That doesn't make any sense, Dad. How can I die if I'm already destroyed?'

'We need to get you in the bath, my man.'

'Can we battle?'

Sigh.

'If you wash your hair.'

We washed his hair.

'Do you want to be goodies or baddies?' he said.

'It's up to you.'

'I'll be baddies.'

'Fine, where are the figures?'

'They're in the box.'

It had been more than a week since he'd had a bath. Partly I think because he'd scraped his knee and there was a big scab on it. Mainly because of overwork and distraction on our part.

We battled the goodies and baddies. There were only seven baddies in the box, and that included a pirate, who should really have been a goodie. I got some more from a drawer under his bed. Then I noticed it was quarter to nine.

'When they die they splash into the water.'

'*Help! I'm splashing in the water.*'

'He didn't even get hit . . .'

'Dude, it's late, we need to move this along. *Help I'm in the water!*'

'He can swim, he's a turtle.'

'Not being funny, little guy, it's late. If you want strawberries we need to head downstairs.'

'Fine.'

Downstairs, for some reason Jack had *Holby City* on, while looking at his phone. It was very odd, the *Holby City*, lots of acting, quiet sets, well-lit, hard to tell exactly what was going on other than a woman in her twenties with perfect make-up and looking very groomed having a coronary.

Nancy took Ray up and I went into the kitchen and leaned against the fridge, feeling momentarily exhausted, trying to remind myself that every moment with my children will one day feel like a treasure to look back on, knowing it was true, and at the same time not really persuading myself.

Wednesday 8 July

Nancy and I had our first meal out in months. I had called around local restaurants. The sushi place in Willesden was doing takeaway only. Ida's, the family Italian on Kilburn Lane, was closed until further notice. Paradise was closed. Parlour thought they might have a spot if we came *now*, but it was 6.15 and Ray wasn't back from his party, and I hadn't done Joe Wicks. Our best option seemed a gastropub on Chamberlayne Road that was now offering a restricted menu of hamburger, chicken burger, veggie burger, and fries, and mac and cheese. When we arrived Nancy parked up and I sat at a table waiting for help.

'Any sign of service?' Nancy asked when she joined me.

'I think they're on the way.'

Another ten minutes later I realized it might not be a case of simple bad service. I asked a cook behind a row of heat lamps: 'Any menus?'

'No menus. You order on the website.'

'On the website? On our phones?'

'Yes.'

'On our phones, at the table, we order, and they bring drinks and food?'

'Yes.'

Nancy ordered food and I ordered drinks, ticking virtual boxes and pushing virtual buttons. A few minutes later a masked waitress came over with the drinks. An Aperol Spritz for Nancy and an IPA for me. The food came. It was blah. The room, the buttons, the waitress in her welder's mask. The tables too far apart. It was all blah-blah-blah. None of it felt right and we headed back home not that long after we'd left the house.

Thursday 9 July

Ray was up at 6.15 and for obscure reasons already downstairs lurking in the TV room, upset because the iPad hadn't been charged. He grazed on YouTube – videos of the strange family with the dad who probably isn't high on meth but just acts that way – while I tried to watch a cut I'd downloaded of the 'Family' episode of the archive show. 'What can I dooooo?' I tried to get him interested in the live-action version of *Aladdin* with Will Smith. But for some reason the best Hollywood production values and millions of dollars of acting talent couldn't compete with a tweaker dad playing video games in his front room.

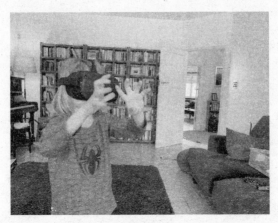

Five-year-old in the metaverse.

Friday 10 July

Zoom quiz last night. We lost again despite having cheated even more aggressively than last time. My current theory is that there are individual teams with members operating out of more than one home, working like cartels, giving multiple answers to a single question. Another working theory is that we have some genius-level quizzers in a cluster in NW10, some of whom occasionally amass more points than are mathematically available from the questions. Or we are just rubbish.

Sunday 12 July

It was the morning and my mum and Michael were coming over. I'd made a quiche with roasted tomatoes and parmesan, using a BBC recipe that required you to make the pastry from scratch. I had to 'blind bake' the pastry case, an expression I'd heard but couldn't quite recall what it meant. I read further down. You had to use 'baking beans'.

'Oh yeah we've got those,' Nancy said.

She brought out a tub of 'ceramic baking beans'.

'Seriously? We've got those weirdo baking beans.'

'*Beads*,' she said. 'Not *beans*.'

It did in fact say *beans* on the tub but I didn't press the point. In the end, I overbeat the egg and forgot to prick the pastry case, plus it was possibly not 'biscuit brown' but pale beige, even though I'd kept it in for the upper limit of the suggested time – thirty minutes total. Whatever. I took it out and put the egg mixture in. When that had cooked it had risen almost like a soufflé.

When they arrived, Mum and Michael again came down the side passage and sat outside on the deck as I fussed with last-minute things like making a salad and putting out cutlery. They'd brought champagne for Nancy's and my wedding anniversary, which is tomorrow.

'But you mustn't feel you must open it,' my mum said.

I drained my coffee, then we opened the champagne and caught up. My mum had had a fall earlier in the week. Walking down Finchley Road, she had stumbled over a paving stone and bruised her knee and elbow and possibly broken a rib. We moved on to other subjects, like anti-vaxxers and statues coming down, then when my mum was out of earshot, Michael, maybe feeling we hadn't talked enough about it, said, 'Yes, it was pretty serious, the fall.'

'It sounds it,' I said.

'It's the fourth one she's had.'

'Wow. That's worrying. I knew there had been two.'

Later, I said to my mum, 'I didn't realize there had been four falls.'

'Only two,' she said, 'and don't believe what he says about me and the tramp.'

'He didn't say anything about you and a tramp.'

It turned out after she'd fallen, at Finchley Road, a drunken homeless man had offered to help, and she'd been so shaken and upset she'd told the homeless man to 'fuck off'.

'I'm not proud of it. Really it was Michael's fault for not fending the man off.'

'Quite right,' Michael said. 'I should have tackled him to the ground.'

'You should have hit him over the back of the head with a black-jack,' I joked.

We ate the quiche and after lunch I inflated the paddling pool, since the weather was warm. Mum and Ray read some of his Kipper and Biff books. Then I threw the Aerobie for Jack as he did flying jumps into the paddling pool and Michael filmed using the phone's slow-motion function, calling out encouragement like a spectator at a bullfight. 'Bravo! Well done, Jack! *Ándale!*' When they went, around five, I had the feeling of a visit well spent. Afterwards my mum sent a message saying: **I didn't realize how much I missed you all.** I texted back: **We loved seeing you!**, meaning it, hoping we would be able to do it again soon, knowing that these times are precious, and that the children are storing up memories for a life-time, and a future when they too will be old and will think back to an afternoon with their grandparents in the garden in Willesden.

Monday 13 July

'On this day eight years ago Mummy and Daddy got married,' Nancy explained to Ray.

'That doesn't make sense,' Ray said. '"This day eight years ago."'

'Well, it's like your birthday. On the same day every year.'

I had – gulp – forgotten, despite my mum bringing the gift of champagne only yesterday. I nipped out after lunch and bought some English sparkling wine and chocolates and a card. We ordered sushi. I was drinking bourbon and orange juice and may have overdone it a shade. We watched an episode of *Watchmen*. It's set in an alternate present, in an America where superheroes are real but morally flawed and a racist alt-right terrorist underground has infiltrated the police. Society's best hope for unity is the creation of an otherworldly enemy, which arrives in the form of torrents of squid creatures which rain from the sky. The show was made more than a year ago but the squid creatures struck me as an eerily prescient metaphor for Covid.

Afterwards I went upstairs and had six or seven goes at recording an announcement of an upcoming corporate on my computer. I was conscious of not being completely sober, but imagined that with some concentration I could pull it off. 'I am so excited to be part of the Widgets & Co Audience with Louis Theroux . . . Expect fun and intelligent conversation . . . And yes I WILL be answering questions about Joe Exotic.' I was slurring quite a bit, so I kept trying again. 'I was a bit tired when I did this,' I wrote to my agent, hesitantly finding the keys on my keyboard. 'Happy to do it again tomorrow if it's unusable.'

Wednesday 15 July

On the *Today* show: masks will be compulsory in all shops from Wednesday next week. But masks not compulsory in places of work due to most people working alongside the same people, ergo in a bubble. There was mention made of a surge of cases – in Greater Manchester I think – it was hard to hear over the kettle. And the possibility of a further spike this winter – that the 'worst may be yet to come'.

The kids are in their last week of school – well, homeschool – before the summer break. Today was Ray's last day in reception. Nancy did drop-off and snapped some shots of Ray going into class with his friends, camera-shy Ray trying to hide behind one of his teachers. A few weeks ago he brought home a socially distanced class photo – a montage of single portraits of all the children.

'You're going to be in lime class next year,' Nancy said to Ray.

Jack pretended to snort derisively.

'Lime. That's a weirdo colour.'

'Stop it, Jack,' Nancy said.

'Lime's a nice colour,' Arthur said. 'Pale green.'

At eleven, I told the big guys it was time to go up. Jack was refusing to surrender his phone, refusing to come upstairs, then collapsed halfway up the stairs. 'I just want to lie here for a while,' he said, into his arms.

Thursday 16 July

I got word that the corporate client was being 'tetchy' and not happy with the video I'd done drunk the other night. I had seemed 'unenthusiastic'. 'Maybe you can charm them on the video call,' my agent said.

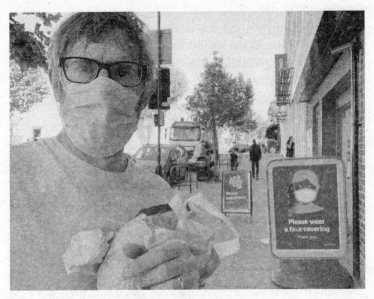

Unexpected item in the bagging area.

Saturday 18 July

'What do you want to do today?' Nancy asked.

We'd been discussing making a day trip somewhere.

'I was thinking Whitstable,' I said.

'Too far.'

'Fine, maybe Margate.'

'Margate's further.'

Ray was lurking in the kitchen having found his way to the iPad.

'I'd just like to go to the beach,' I said.

'Yay, the beach!' Ray said.

'Have you looked at the weather? It's not that warm,' Nancy said.

'It's warm this afternoon. Look. Twenty-three degrees.'

'That's not that warm.'

'You want it *too* warm?'

'You sit on the beach and then what?' Nancy said. 'Even if it is warm, I want to stretch my legs.'

Then, recalling a conversation we'd once had about doing a walk along the upper reaches of the Thames, I said 'What about Cookham?'

An hour or so later, we were parking up on a high street of quaint coffee shops and old pubs and houses with rose bushes out front. We made our way out of the village to an area where there was a car park, a path and a sign telling people to practise social distancing in the fields. We walked on to the footpath, which ran alongside a narrow waterway lined with shrubs in flower and rushes. The sun was going in and out.

'Are those thistles?' Arthur asked.

'Don't know,' I said. 'I'll check the app. *Wild teasel.* It's invasive.'

The app is called *Picture This*. It identifies plants, with almost magical accuracy, after you take a photo of a tiny section of leaf, flower or bark. We carried on along the path, and I checked more plants. About greenery that had once been indistinguishable, I now had a wealth of information: names and alternative names, taxonomy, facts about its uses and its place in folklore. *Hairy willowherb*, a leafy purple flower, was growing in thick bunches. *Purple loosestrife. Broadleaf cattail*, which is a kind of bulrush. The vegetation was like a text that had become legible. Plants with medicinal properties, poisonous berries, hallucinogenic herbs.

'Look, a hot dog plant,' I said to Ray, pointing to the cattail, and I picked one for him. We crossed the creek and walked over to the river, then along the bank. Small boats were sailing and motoring, people were paddleboarding. At the far side was a stretch of well-groomed houses, with broad lawns running down to the river and small covered inlets for their boats. We reached a pub after an hour or a little more, The Bounty. It was only serving drinks, so we pushed on, crossing a railway bridge and reaching a small town called Bourne End where we found a small family-run cafe and ate lunch.

Back home, I thought about the magic of the app. It was extraordinary how much it could reveal, based on a tiny photo. Was it the same with humans, I wondered? Could they identify you from a photo of just your toe nail, if they had enough data? If they couldn't now, presumably all of that wasn't far off, and was that where all the harvesting of data that tech companies were doing was going? Data banks that allowed grey shadowy figures to track you, that would know your health, and predict your behaviour . . . and I guess control you? It was faintly reminiscent of the TV show we'd been watching on iPlayer called *Devs*, about a sinister tech firm that could see into the distant history by taking infinitesimally detailed snapshots of data in the present.

But, if I'm honest, mainly what I was thinking about was the bewitching poetry of the old names. *Wild wormwood, Tansy ragwort, Elmleaf blackberry.* And a lost world of simplicity that they evoked.

Tuesday 21 July

I was driving Ray to Treetops, his summer club.

'Can we check the jar of beer for snails later, Dad?' he asked.

'Of course.'

We'd put out some 'slug pubs' at the weekend – old jam jars in the flower beds, half full of Boddingtons, to lure in and drown the slugs and snails that are overrunning the garden. Partly this was in the interests of pest control, but it was also an 'activity' intended to entertain Ray on a long afternoon. Impatient, I'd picked up a couple of snails and perched them near the edge of one of the jars.

'When do they die?' Ray asked.

'After they fall in. They sort of get drunk and can't get out.'

'Do snails go to heaven?'

'I'm not sure.'

A little later, while I was mowing the lawn, I saw him standing over one of the jars. He was chanting: 'Disappear! Disappear!'

'What are you doing?'

'I want them to go to heaven.'

'Well, it's only their souls that go. So the bodies won't disappear. They'll stay there.'

'Oh.'

Today, Jack appeared from the TV room while Ray ate supper, or rather, he didn't eat supper, since he wasn't happy with the pasta and broccoli he'd been given.

'Has Ray been drowning snails?' he asked.

'No, I haven't,' replied Ray.

'You're a snail *murderer*.'

'No, I'm not!'

'*Murderer*.'

'I'm going to stab you,' Ray said.

'I bet you are. *Murderer*,' Jack said.

'I'm going to kill your soul,' Ray said.

Saturday 25 July

I haven't been writing more because my bones were aching and my joints hurt and I felt grumpy and demoralized. I couldn't do Joe Wicks and every day started and ended with a feeling of anxiety and gloom. I just want to be better or in bed and I didn't feel ill enough to play the sympathy card.

Work has been ongoing on the archive series, a ritual of visits by Tom, me talking about old programmes, trying to draw threads together and make connections, Zoom catch-ups with contributors which we are hoping to use to link material, watching cuts and feeding back notes to editors. The process stretches on and on, partly due to the difficulty of working at distance – the editors are all in their respective homes, which slows everything down – and also the sheer scale of managing four hours of programming at the same time.

Still, we move fitfully in the right direction, with the odd backwards step, and it's a pleasure to see how much in those old shows still holds up and how powerful many of the moments of actuality and emotion still are. A scene in an early episode of *Weird Weekends* about the adult film industry in Los Angeles in which our contributor struggled to get wood on set now has the look and feel of classical verité filmmaking. I stayed in touch with the contributor in question – his porn name was JJ Michaels – and we recorded a long Zoom interview with him. He now lives in Ukraine with wife number six, and a beautiful baby, only a little over a year old, seemingly having found the Shangri-La he was seeking.

Another catch-up call was with Mike Cain. When I'd met him in 1996 he'd been predicting a total breakdown in civil society – he was a 'patriot', a member of a far-right militia community in northern Idaho called Almost Heaven. A gun-rights nut, he believed it was only a matter of time before the New World Order attempted to impose tyranny on freedom-loving people, at which point it would be his obligation to resist, with force if necessary.

Mike never had his showdown with the authorities. He lost his appetite for the fight after his wife left him and after the hordes of well-regulated fellow patriots he imagined were waiting to back him up and defend his house failed to materialize. Then 2000 and the Y2K bug – which he'd seen as a potential trigger point – had passed off without incident, and the sheriffs had closed in. He had fled his house one night to join his wife in Las Vegas. I'd wondered whether Mike might have renounced his beliefs, after all this time, but Mike saw Covid and the hysteria of Coronaland as everything he'd predicted: a fake virus, a sheeplike majority going along with the game plan, wearing their unnecessary masks, and submitting to mass slavery.

But what was most striking when I caught up with him was that the man who'd once fulminated against the federal government, finding nothing to like in any president in living memory, seeing them all as at best dupes and at worst active collaborators in Satanism, was profoundly *in sympathy with* and a fan of Donald J. Trump. A stalwart of resistance and paranoid conspiratorial thinking who had once been ready to take up arms against the feds was now a fare-paying passenger on the Trump Train. It seemed all too revealing of the compass flip Trump represented and the turnaround in the political establishment. Mike the crazy radical, whose moment of bumping up against reality I'd been confidently expecting, hadn't had to accommodate his outlook after all: against the odds, reality had circled around and met Mike's paranoia where it had been for twenty-five years.

The episode of the archive show Mike appears in – which is about 'Belief' – is, in an almost eerie way, a kind of premonition of the Trump phenomenon. In addition to Mike, the second-amendment diehard with a penchant for apocalyptic conspiracy theories, it also features an unscrupulous get-rich-quick guru in Las Vegas, a neo-Nazi family, and an elderly man with weird hair who is in touch with UFOs. Somehow, when Trump pops up at the end of this unlikely cavalcade, it's with a feeling of inevitability, like you've discovered the gene-editing material for the creation of Orange Man.

The 'Dark Side of Pleasure' episode – which looks at the way in which commercial interests have commodified our most forbidden desires, in porn, in gangsta rap, in gambling, in plastic surgery, in prescription drugs – feels, to me, every bit as prophetic, a bitter-sweet requiem for a culture that is in danger of pleasuring itself to death. If anything, the episode which is both most *au courant* but also, for the same reason, the most difficult to get right is the one about crime and punishment, which touches on questions about the racism of the criminal justice system. The George Floyd case is so raw right now, and the animosity against the police is so great from many quarters, that the old documentaries I've made in which the police are seen in a nuanced way, victims after a fashion of structures of inequality which they are required to enforce but which they had no hand in creating, runs a risk of seeming ill-judged in the present moment.

This morning, I had got up early to watch a cut of the archive show featuring clips about crime and punishment and policing. I was vaguely aware of Ray behind me. There was a scene of a man in north Philadelphia being chased down by police and having a gun taken off him, as a crowd gathered and more police arrived.

'So many police!' Ray said. 'And now more police!'

A little later, he said, 'What were the people doing wrong?'

Here we go, I thought. In my head was a phrase I once heard: If the child is ready to ask, they're ready to hear the answer.

'They were selling a kind of medicine that's bad for you,' I said.

'Called drugs. And at first it's nice and then you want more and it can kill you.'

'It's like poison apples, because first they taste good but then they're bad,' Ray said.

It was a little heartbreaking, hearing profound social ills translated into the language of fairy tales, and reflecting how right he was in a way.

Sunday 26 July

We had an arrangement to visit friends at the park. I was still feeling ill but I didn't feel in a position to bail.

On the way, Arthur and Jack were squabbling about their respective haircuts. 'You have a full-on wannabe white roadman haircut,' Jack said. 'And why are you always on TikTok?'

'You go on TikTok, too, Jack,' I said.

'No, I've erased it,' Jack said. 'It's so dead. Plus it's dodgy.'

'What's dodgy about it?' Arthur asked.

'The Chinese government is using it to gather data.'

I felt self-conscious about being ill and mentioned it to Nancy.

'They're going to think I'm bringing Covid. I'll have to just say I've got an upset stomach.'

'Diarrhoea isn't one of the symptoms,' she said.

Jack said, 'Dad's being so dramatic. He thinks he's cool. "Oh, I'm dying of Covid!"'

When we got to the park there was a lot of 'How's your stomach?'

'I'm basically fine now,' I said. 'Something I ate probably.' Later, I googled it, and diarrhoea *is* one of the symptoms.

Are we even in lockdown? Are we coming out of lockdown? *Will life ever be sane again?*

Wednesday 29 July

On the radio this morning, Nick Robinson asking a health expert whether we are at the beginning of a second wave. Reports of rising death tolls in Barnsley, and also on the continent: Belgium, the Netherlands. Should old people self-isolate and keep themselves secluded and safe? Or was it up to everyone, young included, to take measures to reduce contact? Both, the expert said.

Talks are ongoing about whether to make more episodes of the podcast, *Grounded with Louis Theroux*. It is now a month since the last episode in the run of ten – which was the Chris O'Dowd one. Radio 4 are keen. Publicists and agents have been in touch to make people available. A friend is publishing Oliver Stone's memoir, *Chasing the Light*, in the autumn and has offered him up as a guest, which would be a personal thrill and inclines me to want to do a second run, but there are also reasons not to. It takes a lot of time and takes me away from the main business of making TV.

The series is a hit, generating more positive feedback than any TV show I've made in years, which in a way is faintly galling. 'It's been getting me through lockdown' is the phrase of choice. And it only feels slightly odd because I stumbled into doing it, to fill time and to keep busy, and the relative ease of the process makes me a little suspicious of whatever success it's had. I have to remind myself that people tune in for the guests.

It is now my eighth day without Joe Wicks and I think I am still in a slump and I can't believe I have not gone back, but today feels like the first day when I might be on the edge of being able to start back up. Please God. Upset stomach and aches largely gone. Was it Covid?

Thursday 30 July

First Joe Wicks in nearly two weeks. Quick fifteen-minute HIIT. It stands for High Intensity Interval Training. Giddy feeling of reunion, interrupted by kiddie intrusions. Jack wanting my credit-card details to download a new game on the PlayStation for £12.

'It's only twelve pounds, Dad.'

'*Only?*'

'It's a game.'

'What did you do to deserve it?' I heard myself say.

'Mum said I could.'

I checked with Nancy, and it turned out she had approved it.

'*Seriously?*'

'Don't be a Nazi, Louis.'

Winning the fight put Jack in a good mood. 'I believe in women's rights but I'm not a feminist,' he said.

'What alt-right YouTubers have you been listening to?' Art said. 'Seriously bro? What about the gender pay gap?'

'I just think women footballers shouldn't get the same wages because not as many people watch their games.'

'It's a reasonable argument,' I said. 'These questions aren't always easy. Sometimes it's a case of what the market supports.'

After supper, Jack said, 'I'll clear the table if you give me a pound.'

'No, no, no,' I said. 'You don't get paid to clear the table.'

Nancy, to my surprise, disagreed with my position. 'What's the big deal?'

Outraged Louis: 'You don't get paid to do basic chores!'

Jack, angry at what he saw as my obstinacy, and seeing me as the catalyst of the conflict, flared up: 'See what you did? Idiot!'

Now it was my turn to rage: 'Hey, if I pay you a pound, will you *not* call me an idiot?' Warming to my rhetorical device and wanting to continue it, I said, 'If I pay you *ten pounds* will you *not punch me in the face*?'

'You're being weird,' Jack said. 'But yes.'

August 2020

ACTIVITYBOOKMAN

Sunday 2 August

Ray: 'Hey Dad, I've got a joke.'

   Me: 'OK.'

   Ray: 'Why do we have so many pans?'

   Me: 'I don't know.' Thinking: *Because we're in a pan-demic?*

   Ray: 'Because we're *going to Japan*.'

   Me: 'Oh yeah, good joke, Ray!' Thinking: *OK, but we're not in fact going to Japan.*

Monday 10 August

At 10 a.m. a Zoom call with Joe Wicks. It was the first Zoom call I've set up myself. I've had to take out a subscription to the service, otherwise the calls only last forty minutes. Joe and I have been DMing back and forth about the possibility of working together through Mindhouse on a documentary or a series about him and his mission. Joe's brother Nikki, who's his manager, was also on the call. Glimpsing my bookshelves and cupboards, which Nancy recently had repainted, Joe said, 'I know that colour. It's Elephant's Breath. We've got the same colour in our house.' I had no idea our cupboards were Elephant's Breath and couldn't help admiring his surprising level of esoteric colour knowledge.

'To do anything with Joe would be an honour,' I said. 'To spread the word about fitness.'

'We've had other offers,' Nikki said. 'But we like where you're coming from. I think you get it because you're on board with the mission.'

'I am *so* on board with the mission,' I said, thrilled and feeling maybe the way young squires felt when they'd been knighted by King Arthur. 'It's changed my life.'

'Great call with Nikki and Joe,' I said to Nancy afterwards. 'Do you know, he recognized our paint colour on sight? Elephant's Breath.'

'That's not Elephant's Breath,' she said. 'Elephant's Breath is Farrow and Ball. Ours is just a grey they mixed up at Homebase.'

Tuesday 11 August

Searingly hot – our second consecutive 'tropical night', which apparently means over 20°C. More evidence of climate change, were it needed. I sweated so much in the night I think I lost ten pounds, waking up the human version of a raisin, all my liquidity squeezed, desiccated and excreted.

I cycled into town for a story meeting on the Jeremy Bamber project, then had to pedal off again to a *Mail Weekend* magazine photo shoot to promote the archive show – which is now called *Life on the Edge*. I was met in a big posh hotel in Spitalfields by a woman called Vicky. She seemed jittery. She was wearing a mask and said, 'I haven't worked for five months. This is my first job.'

'Should I be wearing a mask?' I had one in my backpack.

'I don't know. I have to. I have to wear full PPE.'

We went upstairs – the lifts had signs saying no more than three people – and in a hotel suite Vicky put on a secondary shield guard over the mask she already had on.

There was photographer Neil, assistant Will, picture editor type person Isabel and a stylist called Grace. Everyone was sweating. Vicky kept checking herself, stressed and adjusting to the new demands of life on Planet Covid. In the bedroom, the implements of prettification were laid out. She had a tube of ointment or gel or face paint which she was waving. 'I'd normally put this on my arm but I can't do that now . . . I feel like Darth Vader in this.'

We went up on the roof, which looked out over the London cityscape, the looming skyscrapers of the financial district and the monuments of big business and empire all arrayed around us. The sun was beating down. Neil the photographer's laptop had over-heated and fritzed out. But we were all aware of there being a job to do, and maybe conscious that none of us had been out much for four or five months, and this was our chance to get back into the groove.

'Square on,' Neil instructed. 'Foot up here. *Life on the Edge*, so you're on the edge.'

Vicky was still wearing her Darth Vader gear, popping over every now and then to pat down tufts of hair and blot my forehead.

'You're outside now, I think you're OK,' I said.

'No, because I'm getting close to you . . . social distancing,' she said.

We tottered around the baking rooftop. More photos – the heat almost surreal in its intensity. With my foot on the edge of the building, illustrating the concept, I was mainly aware of the need not to fall *off* the edge, swoon and swallow dive to an early demise. Then we made our way downstairs to a conference room, where we did more pictures, with a huge paper backdrop rolled out. 'Just keep moving. Lots of different faces,' Isabel said. Neil put some music on. 'What would you like to listen to? Any requests?' I did my best to be game, moving my face around, eyes wide, frowning, smirking, looking bemused, then jumping up and down, doing karate kicks and twirls. An in-person photo shoot. This was my life going back to normal. Which in this case meant me acting like a plonker.

I cycled home.

In the evening, I was putting Ray to bed.

'My back is itchy.'

'Do you want the cream or the lotion?'

'That one.'

'The calamine lotion. Fine.'

'What does it do?'

'It just soothes.'

'What does soothes mean?'

'Makes it feel better.'

A little later: 'My bum is itchy. I think I need some Caroline lotion.'

Wednesday 12 August

Did back-to-back interviews from nine to five at the house to promote the archive series, in a fugue state blur, just speaking and hardly even hearing myself for nearly eight hours.

'Was the Jimmy Savile programme your biggest failure?' asked the man from the *Telegraph*.

Didn't do Joe Wicks and it doesn't feel right. A report that the UK is falling into worst recession on record. More cases in India, an uptick in France. Two thirds of inmates at my old stomping ground San Quentin Prison are infected.

Sunday 16 August

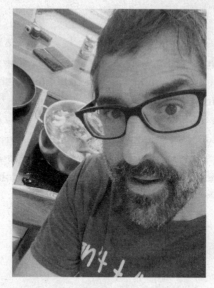

Souper man.

Chania

And so to Greece, where, miraculously, we have managed to repair in the midst of a pandemic, while also observing the relevant protocols. We fetched up on the outskirts of Chania, the ancient Cretan port town, where I am composing this poolside at our rented villa. It is our first family holiday since the onset of Covid – and in fact since last summer.

It had been a scramble to get ready, performing all the unfamiliar tasks of vacating a house that had been our lock-in and hideaway for several months – clearing the garden, emptying the fridge, putting tarps over the bikes. I channelled my low-level travel anxiety into a consuming concern about all the perishables we still had around, spending a precious hour or more that could have been put to use organizing passports and euros improvising a soup out of old green beans, leftover courgettes, and some lettuce and carrots, which I then froze.

We were flying from Gatwick, which was ghostly quiet, and strangely defamiliarized, with the small number of people who were there all in masks. We were all masked-up too of course, except Ray who is exempt, and I found myself scanning the area for signs of non-compliance, in Stasi fashion. Word had come in yesterday or the day before that new rules were in place. People returning from holidays in France were having to quarantine for two weeks. Spain too? Not sure . . . Greece still OK, for now. We ate at a strange notionally health-conscious chain restaurant, where I had a 'picante chicken' wrap. Reasonably certain that a man had not masturbated into it, despite the taste.

On the plane, Ray looked at films on my laptop while simultaneously playing games on my iPhone.

At the Chania airport we picked up our textbook European rental car, new but just that little bit too small and with a tricky clutch, then drove the single-lane Greek highway – where cars pull over into the breakdown lane to let you pass, it seems like madness quite honestly – pulling off to navigate the surface roads, arriving eventually at a scarily steep hillside track which required first gear, and our villa – an ersatz classical structure furnished with little statues of the type you might find at a high-end garden centre. It's built in the Greek style with tiles on all the floors, tight metal doors and window shutters and tiny plastic receptacles for your soiled toilet paper. Not to make a thing out of it, but it always amuses me that a visit to the cradle of democracy and western philosophy involves you fussing with shitty tissues in bins.

We stayed up late, still on UK time. I read *The Digging-est Dog* to Ray. The non-scanning lines bothered me and I tried to change them to make them scan as I went. To help him sleep I'd brought his Google Mini, hoping to get it to play white noise, but every time

I talked to it an unfamiliar Google voice answered, 'I'm sorry. I'm having trouble connecting to the Internet. Please check your network settings and try again.' The voice terrified Ray and he clung on to me in genuine panic.

I ended up in bed with him, after he woke in the night. Then my alarm went off by accident at 7.30 a.m. just as I was having a dream about Seth Rogen and Sacha Baron Cohen – the details didn't stay with me except that in the dream we were friends, and I awoke to a sad reality that I was Rogen-less and barren of Baron Cohen. I dozed on but didn't go properly back to sleep and at around 8.30 Ray, who'd been shifting and sighing, said, 'I want to go downstairs.' I said, 'It's still early,' and in fact the shutters were so effective it was hard to tell, but he shifted and sighed some more, and I said, 'OK, we can go down.'

I was mindful of not wanting to wake the other two boys. I thought Ray might want to watch something on the computer but he reached for an activity book Nancy had bought at Gatwick and we went outside and sat at a marble table by the pool and did colouring. It was called *Funny Faces*: there were sticky-backed eyes and mouths for placing on the faces of monsters and vampires that came with the book. I felt dazed and gormless, and underslept, but I was taking pleasure from his enjoyment and the fact that he wasn't just slumped in front of YouTube watching another family playing video games.

Pointing to one of the pictures, Ray said, 'I just realized that guy's evil because he's got a cobweb up here.'

As we coloured, I was trying to read the *New York Times* on my iPhone – stories about a new book by Kurt Andersen and an article by the op-ed columnist David Brook about the causes of the Trump phenomenon – while also concentrating on colouring inside the lines of a vampire in the *Funny Faces* book.

Nancy came down after an hour or so. Ray and I coloured some more, and then, around ten, I drove into town, winding down, past olive groves and rough cement walls with rebar poking out, on a dirt road with ruts and cracks, into the little town of Lower Stalos. I was trying to find a supermarket, I knew many would be closed, it being Sunday, and also a Greek holiday. I stopped outside Rose Supermarket, which was, despite its name, a rather small mini-mart attached to a hotel and restaurant. The woman inside was blonde and fiftyish with an air of faded glamour. She said her name was Kiki.

'But you can call me "darling", because I call everyone darling.'

'OK,' I said.

'Where you come from?'

'England.'

'England where?'

'London.'

'I love London, where in London you from?'

'West London.' Then I heard myself say, 'Not far from Kensington.' Mainly because I didn't think she would have heard of Kilburn or Willesden or Queen's Park.

She liked this. 'Ah! Kensington – big white houses! You want some wine? You want some tomato sauce? This one I like.' She pointed to a jar of ragù of the sort you can find in most corner shops. 'You looking for somewhere to eat, you come back to my restaurant. The best food in Chania.' The bill for the groceries was huge, more than a hundred euros, and I was aware of being rooked, but not overly worried, figuring it was the price of shopping in a boutique minimart during a Greek national holiday, when all the supermarkets were closed. 'Here, take this, for free,' Darling said, putting a local bottle of wine in my bag. 'See you later, darling.'

'Thanks, Darling,' I said as I left.

Back at the villa, Nancy helped me unload. I was feeling my position vis-à-vis my shopping was solid, especially since, without needing to be prompted, I'd picked up the necessary but easily overlooked basic items like salt and olive oil and also – my ace in the hole – a very large bottle of water, since the water at the house is apparently not potable.

Nancy was silent as we unloaded, but then, finding the salt, said, 'You bought salt? There's a huge thing of salt in the fridge!'

'Oh,' I said. 'Well, salt never goes off.'

'Look!' she said, waving a cylindrical container at me. 'It was in the fridge. That's where they keep it. To keep it dry.'

'OK,' I said. 'Well, the good news is I remembered to get water.'

Ray and Arthur were in the pool. As we put everything away Nancy suggested having brunch outside.

'Sounds good,' I said. 'I could do some eggs.'

I did a quick Joe Wicks, aware I was trespassing on Nancy's forbearance, but I'd also made the point that exercising was part of how I relaxed, and I wasn't going to stop doing it on holiday. I came back down and went out to the marble table by the pool and asked, 'What kind of eggs would you like?' I was harried but also happy, conscious of not wanting to sweat into the eggs, and I ferried food back and forth from the kitchen to the poolside table, then sat down with a plate of toast and Greek tomatoes. Nancy looked up from her eggs, having scrutinized the salt shaker and said, 'Why does it say soda on it?'

'Uh, I don't know,' I said, and then, with a realization: 'Maybe because it's not salt?'

'I thought it tasted a bit weird. I kept putting more and more on.'

'People keep bicarbonate of soda in the fridge, to stop it smelling,' I said. On a roll, and for the sake of the kids, I said, 'Mummy was all, "In Greece they keep their salt in the fridge to stop it sticking!"'

'I never said anything about Greece,' Nancy said.

We spent the afternoon at the beach, then, in the evening, had dinner at a local taverna called Maria's. Walking back to the car I spied Darling sitting outside her shop with some friends. I wasn't sure if she could see me. I angled my head away and scurried over to the other side of the road.

Monday 17 August

Nancy and I got up early to talk about an idea we have been working on for a series about a historic terrorist attack while Ray lounged on my lap. He and I have become slightly obsessed by an app he discovered called *Idle Miner*. You have a team of tiny men who set to work, digging and filling lifts and carts, opening new shafts as you earn more money. You can upgrade your shafts, open new mines – coal, then gold, then ruby – and press different 'boosts'. Your earnings increase in huge increments. First you make millions, then billions, then trillions, then new fictional numbers – 'aa', 'ab', 'ac'. From time to time, the app suggests you push buttons for bonuses and 'special offers' – to multiply the output of your mines – but for these you have to pay ten or twenty pounds *of real money*. The odd thing is, I felt a faint tug of an impulse to spend the money, even though the money you are earning in the game is entirely fictional, and it's all too easy to imagine some vulnerable souls falling prey to the pressure. There are messages that come up saying, 'Remember to take a break!' I googled it. I couldn't find any evidence of people losing their houses after spending all their income on *Idle Miner* – fortunately, or unfortunately, from the perspective of it being a possible story idea.

Tuesday 18 August

We drove into the ancient port town of Chania for some sightseeing, arriving at a square next to the covered market to find there were no parking places. A man with no uniform, possibly some kind of alleged parking manager, who looked like he might be a hustler, said, 'You wait! Two minute! Two minute!'

'I'm not sure about this guy,' I said.

'Dad!'

'He's the parking attendant,' Nancy said.

'I don't see a uniform.'

'Dad thinks he should have, like, an army outfit,' Jack said.

'I think he might be a hustler.'

We were double parked by the side of the road, blocking another parked car. Other drivers were circling around slowly like hyenas, prowling for a space. 'Now you come!' the parking manager said with sudden urgency. I'd been looking at something on my phone, possibly checking my mines on *Idle Miner*, and I hesitated, then pulled off but it was too late. The spot had gone.

'You are SO DEAF!' Jack said. 'Well done, Dad, now we've got no parking space because Dad's deaf.'

Stress levels in the car were high. I drove around the square. Nancy was navigating. 'We're going the wrong way. Go RIGHT!'

'I can't go right, it's no right turn.'

In the back of my mind was a fear of turning down a street that was pedestrianized and taking out revolving postcard displays and fruit carts and men on scooters shaking their fists at me. We seemed to be getting further away from the tranquil seventeenth-century streets of Venetian Chania and into a more modern and rundown part of the city.

'What about here?'

Unexpectedly, we had arrived at a legal parking zone, on the waterfront, and *not* in an area of Cretan street gangs with tattoos and dogs on strings.

Opening the back of the car, I had a muscle memory of taking out a stroller and realized we'd had one the last time we were in Chania a year ago. So this is some kind of passage: our first non-stroller holiday in many years. We walked along the seafront and past the seafood restaurants and the boats tied up at the docks, and the ancient warehouses that bore witness to the Venetian empire that had once been and the cobblestone streets that led back into the interior of the town. We ate lunch, then went for an ice cream, then drove back to the villa. Halfway back, I pulled up outside a Farmakeia. We had an ongoing intimate medical situation that needed addressing.

'I'm not going in to get worm medicine,' Nancy said.

'Seriously? Come on.'

'I'm not. Going in there and pointing at my bum.'

When I came out she said, 'What did you do?'

'I said, "Do you speak English?" and he said "Yes" and I said, "Do you have any worm medicine?"'

Thursday 20 August

After a quiet day at the villa, in the evening we walked up the rutted track, past olive groves and stone walls, to a taverna in the local village. The taverna had a patio which looked across the Cretan hillsides, with the sea in the distance on the horizon. Jack, the gastronaut, ordered snails followed by rabbit. The waiter, who had a wry manner, said, 'I like you.' He was wearing a T-shirt that said 'With This Body, Who Needs Hair'.

'I'll have the volvoi, the Cretan mountain bulbs,' I said.

'OK! You do research before you come here!'

'We had them before. But the other taverna where we had them called them sea bulbs.'

'I don't know. They are volvoi. Mountain bulbs.'

'Grape hyacinth bulbs,' I said.

The mood at the table was growing restive.

The waiter said, 'They are bulbs, how do you say, pickled in vinegar?'

'Yes. Those are the ones. At another taverna they said they grow in the sea.'

The waiter wasn't sure what to say to this.

Afterwards, Jack said, 'Oh my god. So awkward. "*Grape hyacinth bulbs*."'

Monday 24 August

We took a boat trip to a famous Cretan beach called Balos, stopping en route at the Castle of Gramvousa, a fortress built by the Venetians in the sixteenth century to defend their empire from the Ottomans. On board, it was masks at all times and alternate tables only being occupied, in theory anyway, since this was largely disregarded. Before we boarded they shot a small laser gun at our heads to measure temperature.

Wednesday 26 August

We went on another boat trip operated by a company called Beanie's Boats, run by a heavyset sunburned English bloke called Sean, and Beanie, who is his other half.

At lunch, we stopped back at port and ate at a restaurant, and Ray took a loo break. As I stood by the cubicle waiting for him to finish, Ray said, 'Daddy, how do robbers be born?'

'How do you mean?'

'Robbers. How do they be born?'

'Well, they're born like everyone else. Robbing is something people do. Like being a firefighter or an astronaut or a doctor. Except it hurts people.'

'So it's like a job?'

'Kind of, I guess.'

On the drive back to the villa, Nancy was catching up with Twitter.

'Masks on for pupils when they go back to school,' she said.

'Oh, really?' I said. 'Well, as long as they can go back.'

'Ridiculous,' Nancy said. 'Children aren't big carriers!'*

Arthur: 'OK, Karen. "My body, my face!" Seriously, it's not a big deal.'

Nancy: 'It's a big deal to me. It's ridiculous.'

Arthur: 'The masks aren't that uncomfortable.'

Jack: 'It's uncomfortable to me. I like to see my friends' faces.'

After the virtual Democratic Convention last week, this is the week of the Republican Convention, with random Trumps showing up on stage and giving speeches in large numbers like members of the So Solid Crew, vast gestures in an empty venue. Don Jr's

---

* Nancy would later change her position on this, recognizing that children can be carriers and that masks in schools are sometimes a good idea.

partner, a former newsreader, shouted her speech, announcing to an uninterested world that her mother was from Puerto Rico and that her father, from somewhere else, was 'also an immigrant'. It was pointed out that Puerto Rico is part of the USA, ergo not somewhere you can technically immigrate from. I read online that another pair of featured speakers are a husband-and-wife team of personal injury lawyers, Patricia and Mark McCloskey, who literally aimed their guns towards some peaceful BLM protesters in a video that went viral. But my spider senses were telling me that maybe the Trumpers, even without the economy, have found a message that will resonate with enough people – the idea that we are tyrannized by an avalanche of snowflakes and paralysed by nonsensical crypto-anarchist calls to have no police, no prisons, no borders.

Covid deaths in America have been running at around 1,000 a day, according to the *New York Times*, but now are down slightly. Is the virus still spreading? Will there be a second lockdown? Are we going back to 'normal'? I don't want to go back to normal. There was a sense of reassurance in the mass panic. The tranquillity of the gambler who has lost everything and now no longer has to worry about the worst thing happening. Here it is, a world-changing catastrophe to put everything in perspective. Now get on with it. Make some soup or some vegetarian lasagne. Mow the lawn. Make sure you have enough toilet paper or wipe your bum with a magazine and feel like Robinson Crusoe. Work out every day. Get fit. Read a book. Get through the day. Focus on the important things. Let the chaff float away in the breeze.

When we have a barbecue in the evenings at the villa I hop over a wall and scavenge some kindling from the olive grove next to the house. I start the fire, then pile on the coals, then let it settle. Later, when I've cooked and there's just leftovers – uneaten salad, bits of bread, fatty meat – I put them on the fire and watch as it struggles to consume the wet tomato, the damp watermelon rind, the crusts, but eventually they yield and are incinerated. If I've drunk enough I slip on a couple of bits of non-recyclable plastic and watch them curl and wrinkle and wither into nothing.

Thursday 27 August

We walked up to the taverna in Upper Stalos. We had the same waiter again. He was wearing a T-shirt that said 'Running late is my cardio'.

'I want to order sea urchin,' Jack said.

'I'm not sure you'll like it.'

'Fine, I'll have sea bream because you're making me.'

The kids all ordered drinks – Fanta for Art and Ray and freshly squeezed orange juice for Jack – per a previous agreement earlier in the week about doing it on our last night. In Dad-like fashion, I worried it would take the edge off their appetites and that we would be saddled with leftovers we'd be unable to repurpose, since we are leaving.

Ray, at the end of the table, at work on his pirate activity book, needed help adding the number of coins in a chest.

'How many is it, Dad?' he said.

'Well, what is four plus three?'

'I don't know.'

'Try using your fingers. Four . . . five . . .'

'AAH! JUST TELL ME!'

Earlier he had been saying he would like to have a YouTube channel.

'What would your name be?'

'Ray5000,' he said without pausing. 'I could be on it with you like the KidCity family.'

'But what would my name be?'

'ActivityBookMan,' he said. I might have hoped for a catchier name but took it as a compliment.

The waiter came back. He asked about my job. Was I a TV

journalist? Someone at the restaurant had recognized me last time I was here.

'Yes, I'm a TV journalist in the UK.'

'I don't recognize you. I apologize.'

'No problem.'

'Because this woman was excited. She say, "Oh my god, oh my god!"'

'Well, that's nice to hear.'

'But I'm sorry I don't know you.'

'Don't worry.'

'So I just ask to find out.'

'Well, don't worry, I'm not doing an undercover investigation about Cretan restaurants.'

I've used versions of this line many times over the years, usually eliciting at the very least a chuckle or an indulgent smile, but on this occasion it was clear the remark was a misfire. He looked serious and put his hand on his chest and made a reply of the utmost earnestness, along the lines of: 'Please. I assure you, we have nothing to hide.'

'Ha ha! Yes, of course,' I said.

When he went, Jack and Arthur said more or less in unison, 'Oh my god, Dad! So cringe!' 'Just don't, Dad.'

'It's bonding through humour, guys. There is no problem here.'

'You freaked him out. Oh my god!'

I was feeling under attack and I went outside for a minute to look at Twitter and have a moment to myself.

Friday 28 August

This morning we realized that while we were at the restaurant Ray, aged five, had somehow opened a TikTok account and posted several videos of himself online. One of them already has more than a thousand views and fifty likes. It shows him self-shot from below, opening and closing his mouth wordlessly like a carp, and then saying, 'Blah blah blah I like Roblox.'

'I don't think five-year-olds are allowed to post on TikTok,' I said.

'Obviously!' Jack said. 'You have to be thirteen to have an account.'

Ray was thrilled. Beneath his videos were mainly negative comments. Then one poster had written: **don't hate on the kid he just be vibin**

Saturday 29 August

Back in London. House in disarray. Spent a day trying to get on top of it. Defrosting a fridge that was covered in ice. Drifts of autumn leaves around the front door. Piles of luggage and laundry. In the evening I watched *Salvador* with Nancy, as prep for my interview with Oliver Stone – the second run of *Grounded* is happening. The movie took me back to 1986 when it was released and I'd watched it at boarding school, on the last night of term, to celebrate. It was the custom for boarders to lay in tins of Carlsberg Special Brew from the local offy and get drunk, and, later on, vomit into bins around the school premises. Or maybe that was just me. *Salvador* still had a beguiling authenticity. Ragged and a little patched together but full of heart.

Sunday 30 August

Mowed the lawn. Tried to address the acorn situation in the back garden. Took Ray to Roundwood Park for a long session of 'commentating' as he clambered around in the playground. 'This young contender, this plucky newcomer who has defied all expectations with his tenacity and his can-do, will attempt the ultimate challenge . . . going up the slide on his hands and knees . . .' I was feeling listless and aware I was phoning it in. There were posted instructions to 'leave the area if it's too crowded' and 'wipe yourself down after using the rides'. A couple of rides had been decommissioned – including the large round swing – though it was hard to tell if it was due to Covid restrictions or normal vandalism. After the playground session, we walked over to the fenced-in area that houses the yellow Wicksteed exercise machines and for a while Ray amused himself on those, swinging and pumping iron, though they were far too big for him, while I made noises of appreciation.

Riots continuing in America. Consensus that the unrest is playing into Trump's hands. Veteran US news anchor Dan Rather tweeted that the Republican message is that only Trump can save America from Trump's America.

Judging from the news and Twitter, the US appears to be unravelling.

September 2020

THESE DAYS

Wednesday 2 September

There has been a plaintive autumnal music in the skies the last few days, like a fugue for another year gone – brown leaves dancing and whirling in the kerbsides and moisture in the air and low-level silvery light, a sun that seems tired and spent even when it is shining, as though it's been fitted with a lower wattage bulb.

The radio tells us that schools are going back. People are returning to work. Cases of Covid seem to be, not declining, but climbing less rapidly in the US. France's cases are trending up, and so too India's. But movies are back. People are going to see *Tenet*, a Christopher Nolan film about moving backwards through time. Marce wrote on the family WhatsApp that he went to see it. His verdict was: 'srelbboc', which is 'cobblers' backwards.

It's hard to know where everything's heading. Trump was in Kenosha, Wisconsin, defending Kyle Rittenhouse, the vigilante who shot and killed two BLM protesters. He claimed that antifa and BLM figures are stocking up on tins of soup as ammo to throw at enemies. A report on the news said that, according to a new book, Trump had 'a series of small strokes' in 2019 and was hospitalized in Walter Reade medical centre in NYC. He is denying it, but the phrase 'Strokeahontas' was trending on Twitter. Many jubilant reflections on the neatness of the satirical moniker, and a handful of others decrying it as racially insensitive to Native Americans.

I spoke to Marce.

'I stay off Twitter,' he said.

'It's like a Wild West saloon,' I said. 'Chairs flying through the air.'

'I don't even read the papers. It's too triggering.'

'Snowflake,' I said.

'Sorry not sorry.'

'Libtard,' I said.

Arthur spends his evenings upstairs watching movies with his friends remotely. Jack watches gamers on YouTube. Ray lives on his iPad.

Thursday 3 September

We had an office day in Soho. With certain restrictions, we can meet at a workplace, and so for one day a week we have access to a couple of rooms on Berwick Street. It's a little odd, the feeling of it being temporary and provisional, and sniffing around each other in unfamiliar Covid-safe ways. We had a Zoom catch-up with BBC commissioners about ideas I might be able to present in the UK. Police access, with me embedded in a police force in a high homicide area? A Pupil Referral Unit, getting to know the troubled kids and their home lives? Something more celebrity focused? There is also a feeling that the success of *Grounded* may present a model for a television format. I still have reservations, wary of getting back into the way of working we had when we made the *When Louis Met* series in the early 2000s. Stressful negotiations about access. A feeling of being parasitic, feeding on the life and success of another person. And requiring – as we did then – days and days of their time for filming to get what we need.

But we have to be realistic, and with travel restrictions still in place US ideas aren't looking makeable anytime soon, with the possible exception of the Joe Exotic one since it relies heavily on archive and should only need a week or so on location. The other option – of making slice-of-life documentaries in which I'm immersed in gritty subjects in the UK – is more achievable, but I'm aware I've made a number of those kinds of documentaries over the last few years and I don't want to weary viewers, and I'd like to stay ahead of expectations a little bit. Also, there is the risk – especially with the police one, but maybe with all of them – of my presence out on location being a distraction. We arrive at a serious crime scene and the bystanders are all saying, 'All right, Louis? Can I get a selfie? What about that Jimmy Savile? You knew, didn't you?'

Monday 7 September

Ray's first day back at school.

'How was it?'

'Medium,' he said.

'OK,' I said.

'Four bad things happened to me,' he said.

What the four things were never became clear.

Last night the first of the archive shows went out. Ratings are 'a bit soft'. Below a million. Yikes. That's low. What happened? 'People watch on iPlayer nowadays,' I said to Nancy, not totally believing my own damage control. The reviews were mainly good. Well, good-ish. Three stars in the *Guardian*. 'A clip job . . . but what clips they were.' The reviewer would have liked more exploration of 'process' and 'unintended potential complicity'. There was also this: 'Disingenuousness has always been part of the Theroux brand – or a tool of the trade, for this is not a criticism.' Four stars from the *Telegraph*. 'An intriguing catch-up.' And the obligatory reference to the 'endearingly gawky filmmaker'.

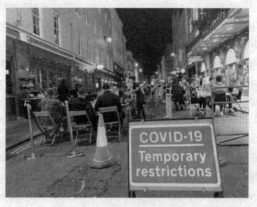

Socially distanced Soho.

Wednesday 9 September

Arthur went back to school yesterday, Jack today.

In the evening Nancy and I went out for a drink and a meal with our TV Insider Friend and his friend, the talented writer and actor Sharon Horgan. The restaurant was called Duck Soup. The Soho streets were laid out with tables, like a Barcelona nightscape. *Maybe this is an improvement*, I thought. *Take back the streets.* I was nervous meeting Sharon. I'm a fan of her HBO series *Divorce*, and was maybe just, in a pathetic way, conscious she was someone I should try to impress, and I was making jokes and chit-chat in a hypomanic way. 'Been making programmes at home! Ha ha! Update shows! You know what it's like. Covid na-na-na-nineteen.'

When she left the table, Nancy said, 'You're trying too hard. Why don't you just be normal?'

'This is my new normal,' I said.

'You're very funny when you're just being natural.'

I was chain-drinking grapefruit margaritas. Afterwards we went to a private members' club, of which our TV Insider Friend was a member. There was a complicated app we had to fill out to come in, involving confirmation emails arriving on your phone, click this, check that. The grapefruit margaritas had rendered me incapable of figuring it out – I couldn't find the buttons to push or the email with the code. Eventually they took pity on us and just waved us in.

Tuesday 15 September

'Mingling' – from the Germanic word 'mingin', which means to knead dough – has been made illegal. The 'rule of six' is in place, as a result of an uptick in cases and the R number going above one again. There are mutterings that it could last until March, which is strange to contemplate, just when things appeared to be starting to return to normal. Home Secretary Priti Patel was on the *Today* show trying to explain the policy but it wasn't clear she understood it completely herself.

The papers complain that we are now in a Stasi-style state where we have to snitch on friends and loved ones if we catch them breaking the rules. You can still go to work – in fact you're supposed to go to work – and go to restaurants, but you can't meet up with people and if you bump into them you're not supposed to spend too long catching up.

Yesterday I was working at half capacity, suffering the after effects of a Sunday afternoon get-together at our house. We had hosted our South London friends, plus their kids, for a last summer hurrah – I'd squeezed lemons for a tequila cocktail called a Juan Collins and we had the paddling pool up, with warm water running into it from an inside tap. It was a beautiful warm Indian summer's day and I was buoyed along by the endorphins from a vigorous thirty-minute Joe Wicks.

By mid-afternoon the Juan Collinses were all *adios*, as were several bottles of wine, and the adult male partygoers were doing running dives into the paddling pool. Ski Mask the Slump God was bumping on the Google Home and I was, in an undoubtedly cringe way, dancing and waving my arms in the air like I just didn't care. I made a fresh round of drinks, then came back out with a tray and stepped into the paddling pool, feeling the need to pontificate on current affairs.

'Elements of the far left have created an open goal for Trump,' I said.

'Exactly,' Musician Friend said.

'Biden seems clinically demented. Did you see the interview with the guy where he was like, "That's like me asking you are you on cocaine" and then he seemed to lose the power of speech?'

Actor Friend called it up on his phone, hanging his arm over the side of the paddling pool so as not to get the phone wet.

'Just search Joe Biden cocaine interview,' I said.

'He looks like he's had a stroke,' Actor Friend said. 'He's just really weird, with all that Botox.'

'And the shiny teeth. At least the Soviets waited until their leaders died before they embalmed them. It's crazy, they rigged the process against Bernie, and now we're all supposed to root for someone who appears to be demented. It's like Defund the Police. What Nancy was saying was they don't actually want no more police. It's about changing the paradigm. It's bad branding.'

I was finding myself extremely interesting. I wanted to get more wine but I also didn't want to get out of the warmth of the paddling pool. By this time the two five-year-olds had grown bored watching the Disney *Robin Hood* and began leaping off the side of the pool and splashing water into our drinks.

When the guests had gone, I laid out some food for the kids, then focused on clearing up, gathering dishes and glasses, and doing the third dishwasher load. I suspected I might be over the line because I noticed I was playing *Nina Simone at the Village Gate* on repeat on the Google Home, which is generally a sign. I put on some Velvet Underground – 'Femme Fatale' – and some Nico, and thought what a shame it was I couldn't go on *Desert Island Discs* again and choose different records. I'd heard that David Attenborough had been on three times. Who knew? Maybe one day. I'd definitely choose this one. *Don't confront me with my failures.* As I sang along with the music I reflected that I couldn't really be that drunk since I was still capable of thinking I shouldn't get too drunk, and I was only topping up my drink in very small increments, plus it wasn't that late.

At 9 p.m., when the latest instalment of my *Life on the Edge* series came on TV, I ducked into the front room and watched the beginning with Nancy and – surprisingly – Arthur. It was the first time I'd ever been with him for one of my programmes going out. He lay on a bean bag and looked at his phone.

I noticed I had double vision.

'You're drunk,' said Nancy. 'You're doing that squinty thing with your eyes.'

I went back into the kitchen and did some more tidying. Then, thinking I should probably catch up on some work, I watched an episode of *I May Destroy You* as prep for a scheduled conversation with Michaela Coel.

The next morning I awoke melancholic and sheepish, with almost no recollection of what had been in the episode of *I May Destroy You* – aware I needed to probably watch it again.

'No drinking tonight,' I said to Nancy.

'I told you you were drunk,' she said.

'Well, you were right.'

It feels like we are back in some cover version of lockdown; same lyrics, different arrangement.

Friday 18 September

On the *Today* show this morning, I heard Van Morrison has released three new songs protesting lockdown and the response to the pandemic. A Covid-sceptic grudge-list set to the chord progression of 'Brown Eyed Girl'. (It's not actually that.) By coincidence, we have tickets to see Van in a few days. Maybe, instead of an evening of mystical Celtic minstrelsy, it'll all be protest songs about 5G masts and flu deaths being chalked up to Covid.

News that the New Year's fireworks in London cancelled. Rumours of a further lockdown.

Tuesday 22 September

a.m.

The second wave is here, we are told. Chris Whitty, the government health adviser, has announced we have 'turned the corner', a bad corner, which is a little confusing, since turning corners is usually good. New rules have just been announced saying pubs and bars and restaurants must close at 10 p.m. and there will be no bar service, only table service. Fans will *not* start to return to sporting events in October. Much disgruntlement, especially since Covid scepticism and anti-masker feeling is already running high. There was a demonstration in Trafalgar Square at the weekend with multiple arrests. Case numbers are spiking in France and Spain, too.

On the plus side, there is an amusing viral video of Biden saying in a speech that 200 million people have died from Covid. Which is around 198 million over the real figure.

Morale on the home front is mixed. The kids are seemingly OK. We are relieved to have them back at school. Nancy is worrying about commissions and whether they will still happen with new restrictions in place. Am I still flying to America for the Joe Exotic revisit? Nothing is quite certain.

p.m.

Boris Johnson has announced new measures. We're supposed to be ready for this to last six months. Hospitality industry in crisis. Pubs and restaurants on their last legs. Regional lockdown in the north-east. There are different rules in the different nations and regions. Labour saying the measures are necessary but that the government is incompetent.

Nancy and I were on a Zoom call with Arron. She broke off to answer the phone and then came back, visibly upset.

'Year eights are being sent home. Someone tested positive.'

Jack arrived a little later. He has to self-isolate for two weeks.

Arron said Joe Wicks is back doing three live sessions a week. So there is that.

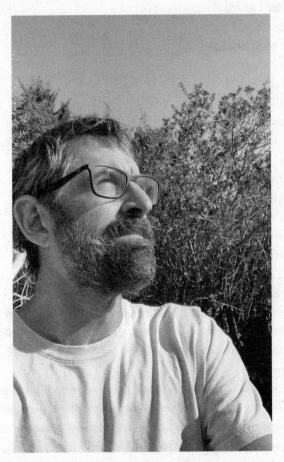

Autumn overgrowth.

Wednesday 23 September

I was considering supper options, scanning a fridge that was close to empty. Finding a single large leek in the vegetable drawer, I started to make a leek carbonara, a Jamie Oliver recipe. Half an hour later I heard Nancy say, 'Fuck!'

'What?' I said.

'Van Morrison!' she said.

'What about him?'

'I totally forgot.'

'Oh! When is it?' I said.

'I thought it was cancelled!' she said.

'You knew it wasn't cancelled because you mentioned it at the weekend.'

'I know but then I forgot. Shit.'

'When is it?'

'Seven thirty.'

It was ten past seven as she said this.

'I don't want to go,' I said. 'I'm not mentally prepared.'

I had my evening laid out in my mind. I was stirring my leek around and thinking it would be at least ten minutes before it was the required soft melting consistency. I'd already mixed my grated parmesan with a large raw egg. I was also warming some Bolognese, for me and Nancy, which would now no longer be needed. It was a nightmare.

'It's too late,' I said. 'There won't be a warm-up. This is a nightmare. I feel overwhelmed.' I was conscious that I was being spineless and wondered whether the long months of not going out and not making arrangements had atrophied my social muscles so that I was no longer capable of fulfilling minor engagements.

'He won't be on at seven thirty,' Nancy said.

'I'm in my pyjama bottoms,' I said. I was thinking: *I've got emails I need to send*. 'What about the leek carbonara?' I asked.

I went upstairs to change out of my pyjama bottoms. An Uber arrived. 'Come on, the Uber's here,' Nancy said.

'You go. I'll be a minute. I'm just dishing up.'

'The Uber is here *now*.'

'I'm dishing up.' I grated parmesan onto the kids' plates.

I called from the car. 'Does the leek carbonara taste OK, Art?'

'Yeah.'

'OK, good.'

Outside the venue – the Palladium – there were temporary metal railings. A man pointed a laser gun at our heads. Inside, the bar was almost empty. There were tubes of crisps, the kind that are basically normal crisps but have names like 'chardonnay vinegar and Etruscan sea salt', and three kinds of chocolate in packets: Munchies, Minstrels, and Revels. There were screens up and masks, of course, and signs: 'Please can you keep your mask on unless you are eating or drinking.'

An old tubby man came out on stage and said, 'Are you enjoying the show so far? The Palladium is a venue with a wonderful history. Fats Domino. Judy Garland. The Beatles. But there is one young man who has never performed here. Until tonight. Ladies and gentlemen, Mr Van Morrison.'

I had never seen Van live before, despite loving his music since I first bought *Saint Dominic's Preview* in 1986. He came out, superannuated and frog-like, but exuding bonhomie, and struck up a song I half-recognized and realized later was 'Three Chords and the Truth'. Then he launched into a jazzed-up version of 'Moondance'. Fair enough. 'Moondance' was fairly jazzy in its original recording, kind of walking bassline and lounge piano. Then there was another jazzy one I didn't recognize. When he lit into 'Saint Dominic's Preview', I thought, *YESSS, it's honky-tonk Ulster folk from here on in . . .* but then he went back into a kind of piano lounge jazz set and then the tubby compere came back out and they traded-off vocals. Whenever the music went too far in the direction of a Hilton Hotel piano lounge track I did a Prosecco run. During one of them, a little down the bar a man nodded at me, then came over and said, 'Louis! Just want to say. We need you. You're a maverick. Keep doing what you're doing.' His name was Peter. He ran a B & B in Broadstairs.

'Thanks,' I said.

Back in the auditorium Van shoo-wopped and dooby-dooed through his last couple of numbers, then ambled off, surrendering the stage to a virtuosic xylophonist, who, having punished her instrument enough, jumped on the bongos, drilling them with astonishing staccato precision. When the set ended, I looked at Nancy and said, through my mask, 'That was great!' We wandered out and were walking up the pedestrianized little thoroughfare that is Argyll Street when a voice called out, 'You want a drink? On me!' It was the man from the bar, Peter. He was with his daughter Lily, a nurse.

'Dad's obsessed with Van,' Lily said.

'Have you seen him a lot?'

'About thirty times,' Peter said.

'How did you rate tonight?'

'Not his best set. He usually does a bit he calls "walking the cat". A medley of his old stuff.'

We ordered four Peronis.

'You like Van?' Peter said.

'I do.'

We exchanged views on his best albums, agreeing that *Veedon Fleece* was the most underrated. Then he asked, 'What about Chet Baker?'

'Love Chet Baker,' I said.

'Better than Miles Davis,' Peter said.

'I don't think even Chet Baker thought he was better than Miles Davis,' I said, and warbled, '*Moon . . . and sand.*'

We had another couple of drinks and talked more about music – a small connection with a stranger, after so little contact with others, wafted along by the good vibes of the gig, Covid-sceptic Van and a rare outing to a live show, after months locked inside staring at screens. As we said our goodbyes, Peter said, 'Come and stay at our B and B.'

'I'd love to,' I said, meaning it, wondering if we'd ever get to do it, and thinking of weekends in Margate and Whitstable and East-bourne, the rain-lashed beauty of the English seaside.

When we arrived home, Arthur and Jack were still up. Nancy and I opened a bottle of red wine and put on 'Caravan' and 'Sum-mertime in England' and we danced in the kitchen in each other's arms.

Friday 25 September

A late autumnal day, dark in the morning. Winter's bony fingers are sliding into the cracks of the house.

The R number is rising. Covid cases going up. Deaths in America over 200,000. Over 40,000 in the UK. Boris is playing out of position: the scrappy and bumbling Churchill karaoke performer having to refashion himself as a technocrat.

Brooding feelings of anxiety that seem to centre on work and the idea that my new series of the podcast won't be any good or that the notion of a chat show – which is still lurking in the background, in conversations with the BBC and other broadcasters – reeks of hubris. I miss being immersed in a story and I find I have a general feeling of disquiet that is hard to pin down. Exercise helps and also alcohol. The two men in my corner are Joe Wicks and Jack Daniels.

Wednesday 30 September

Yesterday it was announced that global virus deaths are over a million. News of the first Trump–Biden debate, a slow-motion car crash by all accounts, with Trump interrupting and badgering Biden. Commentators said Trump lost the plot, even many right-wingers on Twitter seemed muted, and accused the moderator, Fox News's Chris Wallace, of being biased against Trump. In the clips I saw, he looked like Trump-as-usual, doing his soft-voiced snarls of contempt and abuse, 'I don't know about Beau, I know about Hunter, he was dishonourably discharged from the army.' The soundbite that played repeatedly was Biden saying, 'Would you shut up, man?' and also 'You are the worst president in history.' Trump declined to repudiate white supremacism, electing instead to say to the Proud Boys, whose founder and leader Gavin McInnes we have been in touch with on and off over the past year, to 'stand back and stand by.' Much debate about what this catchy formulation – combining two similar-sounding verbs – really means: is it a call to arms or does Trump just like repetition? Given the low bar set for Biden – repeated allegations from his opponents that he is demented, stroke-ravaged and incoherent – he came across as relatively unconfused.

So chaotic and unedifying was the whole affair that there was some speculation that the remaining two debates might be cancelled. Later, it was said that former Governor of New Jersey Chris Christie had been Trump's debate coach, and had told him that Biden, a recovering stammerer, apparently, would be discombobulated by interruption: it might cause his stammer to come back. This was Trump's game plan.

On these shores, rumours circulate that Boris is underpowered and disorientated and suffering from 'Long Covid' – supposedly it takes months, even years to shake, debilitating those who catch it, rendering them incapable of exertion, making them weak and breathless, like ME. In a speech, he mis-explained the latest rules on social interaction. He is said to have lost his 'élan' and his 'buoyancy'.

I had a crazy beginning of the week, doing three Zoom interviews more or less back to back – a chat with the visionary musician FKA Twigs on Monday, a conversation with celebrity ex-Scientologist Leah Remini on Tuesday evening, and then this morning my one-to-one with writer and actor Michaela Coel, whose series *I May Destroy You* has been one of the hits of the pandemic.

I'd been nervous before the Michaela interview, as I am before most of my *Grounded* conversations, but with her in particular, obviously because I'm a fan of the work and wanted it to go smoothly, but also because I was conscious of how *in demand* she is at the moment and aware that her doing my podcast, with all the offers that must be brimming in her inbox, was a huge favour and vote of confidence, and I didn't want to disappoint with anything that was subpar.

I'd watched *I May Destroy You* on catch-up, after multiple recommendations, and was relieved to find it did not disappoint. It features a series of sexual encounters that run the gamut from out-and-out assaultive to something more ambiguous, confused hook-ups and trysts between people who are in different ways not seeing each other clearly. It is, among other things, a kind of anatomy of how sex takes place for millennials, via apps and phones, and so for me had an almost ethnographic interest, which isn't to undersell its visual flair and the awkward comedy that lifts it above the realm of grim. Above all, what felt special was the feeling that raw, confronting issues were considered by a guiding intelligence that was magnanimous and able to see things from multiple angles and interested in the awkward and inconvenient grey areas.

The chat had been arranged via her agent and my producer. She'd been away, which delayed it. Other *Grounded* interviews I've done have run on to two or even three hours. I was told Michaela only had an hour and a half, which, given they all end up being around an hour after editing, seemed achievable. Then, a few minutes before the appointed start time, a leaf blower started up outside, which threw me. But then we got going and I realized that even with all her success she is at heart, mainly, a curious person, simple as that sounds: someone interested in life and its contradictions, grappling in the same way we all are with what life looks like in a world where sexual opportunity sits alongside victimization and where the lines of oppression aren't always as clear as we might ideally like.

A lot of the conversation ended up centring on race and in particular – for some reason – the way in which some white men and women fetishize black sexuality. She mentioned a white male friend of hers who had said he preferred dating black women because they had 'more soul'. My reply was along the lines of, it's a short step between 'more soul' and 'natural sense of rhythm', and one of my few regrets afterwards was that I didn't have the presence of mind to mention the ongoing civil suit brought against Harvard University by students of Asian heritage, on the ground that they have been systematically discriminated against, being marked down on their candidate profiles for 'lack of personality'. It had struck me as a kind of symmetrical racism: their case was that they were being viewed as having *too little soul*.

By the end, we had covered her Ghanaian heritage, her upbringing in the City of London in the shadow of the financial district, her own personal experience of sexual assault, and the whole topic of her having a moment centre stage, with calls coming in from Steven Spielberg and Donald Glover. When I offered to wrap things up at ninety minutes, she said she still had time, and I asked about her current dating situation, a question she batted away, and what she was working on now, and she mentioned the phenomenon of 'post-writum depression', a phrase I enjoyed, and soon after that Paul the producer jumped back on and we arranged the transfer of audio files from her end to ours.

It was midday when I finished and I came downstairs and Nancy was there, happy because she had just heard that Channel 4 had commissioned our series with Alice Levine, called *Alice Levine's Sex Odyssey*, but also harassed due to a sudden rush on our treatment about snooker players in the 1980s, which she wanted me to look at. I scanned it and gave feedback, but grumpily, correcting small errors of phrasing and punctuation, and feeling overwhelmed by how much there was to do.

'Some of this is gibberish,' I said.

'I told you it needed work.'

'Is it really the best use of my time? It's like the CEO of Ford coming down to the factory to screw the lug nuts on the cars.'

I actually said this, and it went down about as well as you might expect, leading to a short but lively exchange of views. A little later I was doing a Joe Wicks to blow off some steam – fifteen minutes, hardcore, forty on twenty off, with five rounds of burpees at the end – when my phone started buzzing with WhatsApp messages. My niece, at university in the Midlands, had tested positive for Covid, along with all her housemates, but with no symptoms.

Afterwards I made supper – beef steaks for the kids and quiche for me and Nancy – and then I hit the Bulleit hard – maybe from the relief of having three more episodes of the podcast wrapped up in the last three days. I watched a Frankie Boyle stand-up special – *Excited For You to See and Hate This* – on my computer. Nancy was in the front room watching her own programmes. I was properly drunk by now, guffawing like a deranged person, like a patient in purple psychosis who suddenly sees the grand plan. The comedy was macabre but thoughtful, the kind of humour that walks a dangerous line between offensiveness and intelligence. 'Daring the void', as Adam Parfrey once put it; jokes that you couldn't justify except *as* jokes, even though, as someone once said to me, 'there's no such thing as a joke'. The darkness was uncomfortable, which added to it, and by the end I was no longer trying to understand why it might or might not be OK but just laughing.

The lights in the kitchen were off and the room was dark and I had my headphones on and later I was conscious of how I must have looked, inebriated, face lit by the screen, laughing away on my own at apparently nothing.

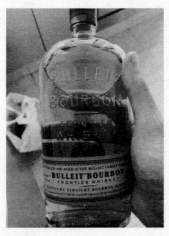

Hello, friend. Are you ready to dance again?

October 2020

CURIOUS AND
UNUSUAL DEATHS

Thursday 1 October

Arthur is in the top bedroom now, which I was using as a study before. I've taken Nancy's study, which is above the kitchen, with only a thin ceiling in between, meaning that when I work in the evening and there are people downstairs, mainly Jack, I can hear DigDat and Headie One and AJ Tracey coming through the floor or the buzz of the NutriBullet making smoothies.

Jack is still at home, notionally home-learning, though we wonder how much home-learning is happening.

This morning, Ray was up at 6.55, his voice calling out, 'Daddy!'

'I'll lie down with you for a minute, OK? Because it's still early.'

That lasted about fifteen minutes. I was feeling rough, fogged-out, my kidneys marinaded for twelve hours in Bulleit bourbon. I came downstairs with Ray. He seemed tired too, watched KidCity on YouTube while I washed up and unloaded the dishwasher and licked my booze-soaked wounds. Nancy came down, and the big boys.

'You are somewhere else,' Nancy said.

'I'm right here.'

'What's going on with you at the moment?'

'Nothing is going on with me.'

• • •

Was anything going on with me? I wasn't sure. Possibly I was fine. Possibly I wasn't. It was hard to know. Was it wrong to drink quite so much? What if you could still function and you enjoyed it and most of the time you felt OK? Was I hiding? Was I dulling the pain? Was it weird that I didn't have more insight into what was going on or was that what most men were like? The radio was saying there were further local lockdowns in the north-east, and in Liverpool too. But college students could come home for Christmas. Even if they found a vaccine in the spring, the radio said, it would take years for life to return to normal. Whatever that meant. And, in fact, what about this assumption that we should return to a normal that involves forest fires literally the size of Uruguay and mass extinction? We were all so keen to save humans and sure humans are great – I love the Sistine Chapel and I happen to be married to a human – but did we really deserve quite so much consideration given that we were rampaging around the planet in Hummers and selling avocados in stupid plastic packaging and giving gift bags at children's parties that ended up in the guts of sperm whales thousands of miles away? *Wah wah wah! The coronavirus! Wah wah wah! We need more humans to fuck up the planet so we can watch YouTube and dolphins can die choking on a mini Rubik's Cube.*

The fog lifted over the course of the day, helped along by a vigorous twenty-minute Joe Wicks. As I came out of the shower, the doorbell rang. It was one of the neighbours.

'Have you signed the petition?' she asked.

'What's it about?'

'The 5G mast they want to build at the end of the road.'

'I'm going to be honest with you,' I said, surprising myself with my directness. 'I don't believe it's going to fry my brains and I'd quite like the faster internet.'

'Sure, OK,' she said. 'So I guess that's a no?'

Friday 2 October

Trump has coronavirus. The news came in about 5 a.m. London time and it was like the radio was scrambling to keep up. It seemed both the weirdest and the most predictable twist in the whole saga of 2020. *Of course* he's got the virus. The reality-distortion field he projects, so powerful against the media, against his friends and his enemies and the economy and maybe even foreign despots, is useless against a remorseless scrap of self-replicating DNA.

He'd caught it from his political adviser Hope Hicks, they thought – or at least they'd tested him after she tested positive.

I said to Ray at breakfast, 'Trump's got the coronavirus.'

'Yay,' said the five-year-old, and raised his arms.

'Well, we don't really want people to be sick. Even Trump.' [Pause.] 'Except I do kind of want him to die.' The words were out without me even being aware of it. 'I don't want him to die. Of course, I don't.'

Saturday 3 October

Nancy's birthday is tomorrow and to celebrate I arranged for a hotel stay for the two of us in Brighton, while Nancy's mum takes care of the children at her house in Kent.

I'd got up at 8.40 feeling rough following a boozy dinner with local friends and late-night vodka-fuelled arguments about the efficacy or otherwise of lockdowns. Advertising Friend, who is a recovering socialist turned lockdown sceptic, kept saying to Nancy, 'I'm really impressed with you,' after she voiced lockdown-sceptical views about the pandemic and how much spreading was really happening in schools, while Eco-Photographer Friend was discoursing on the lessons to be learned about solving climate change, which involved – I think; I was sozzled at this point – recognition that at times of adversity humans have a track record of pulling together, cooperating and finding solutions

'The key word is altruism,' he said.

'I'm not honestly sure that's how it works,' I said, offering my own more or less apolitical two cents' worth. 'You could just as easily make the case that a crisis brings out the worst in us. What is it Brecht said? Food first, then morals. Something like that anyway. Is that my vodka?'

I dropped Ray off at Stagecoach, his Saturday morning drama workshop, then, realizing I'd left my jacket at the friends' house the previous night, I went round to pick it up – I wouldn't have cared except it had a parking ticket in the inside pocket which I needed to pay. Late morning we all drove down to Nancy's mum's, getting stuck in a traffic jam caused by flooding caused by incessant rain caused by climate chaos caused by humans. The jam was so horrendous – cars were static; massive puddles everywhere – it seemed to license us to ignore the normal rules of road safety and do whatever we could to escape, but the stress of the entire mis-adventure and the claustrophobia of the car catalysed a fist fight between Jack and Arthur, until Nancy screamed at them and I scrambled back mid-journey to separate them – we were driving seventy-five down the motorway by now and I was doing yoga-style slithering around the vehicle to wrestle my children away from each other. I slept a bit more in the car, which perked me up a little, though I still sounded husky and dark brown when I arrived.

'Has Louis got a cold?' Nancy's mum asked.

'No, he's just hungover,' Nancy said.

I'd made a reservation at the Grand and a restaurant called the Flint House. We checked in – wearing masks, and there were hand pump stands about the place. I had a shower and then like lovers in a dream we talked and talked and actually interacted with each other in a way that didn't involve crisis management or resentment but instead pleasure and getting to know one another again.

We went out to eat, us both in our masks walking along the dark rain-slicked streets of Brighton. I'd gone to a bit of trouble to secure the various reservations, googling, checking ratings on Tripadvisor, phoning, emailing, conscious that if I put my full name at the end of my messages it might smooth the way a bit. Most of the places I'd had my sights on were full up but I'd eventually found somewhere and I was feeling some combination of smug and relieved, like I'd dodged a death sentence or passed an important exam – the Nancy birthday finals. We made our way through an area called The Lanes, a labyrinth of narrow alleyways, which was like a location from *Pirates of the Caribbean* where miscreants are press-ganged into sea-borne servitude. We ate. There was a 10 p.m. curfew and we made our way back at 9.45 through huddles of young students, and lay and drank some champagne I'd ordered as part of the room package, and Nancy dozed.

Monday 5 October

Trump is apparently out of hospital, still presumably infected with corona, and gallivanting around the streets outside Walter Reed Medical Center in Maryland. I didn't want him to die because he's a fellow human and that would be wrong, but it's a little discouraging to see him bounce back quite so easily.

Sunday 11 October

I had a bad few days due to some kind of GI infection, a bacillus nestling in my small intestine making me weak and listless. Any food I managed to eat came back up into my mouth in small gobbets a few hours after I ate it. When I did a shit the toilet bowl looked like a Pollock painting. But what mainly worried me was the need for sleep and an inability to work in any concentrated way. It had started on Tuesday. I'd woken up thinking I was just hungover from a late-night pile-up involving two gin and tonics, some red wine and a strong Bulleit and orange juice concoction which steamed in at about 11.30.

The next morning, after the kids had gone off to school, I did a fifteen-minute Joe Wicks to try to shake myself into some kind of health, but towards the end I was sweating more than usual, feeling nauseous and I realized I might be coming down with something, and I had to lie down.

The following day, I was scheduled to interview Ruby Wax for the new series of *Grounded* and thought about postponing due to illness, but I knew that might cause issues of its own, since there is already a fraught emotional atmosphere over the encounter. The pretext for the booking – apart from her being a very funny TV presenter with a track record of interviews with high-profile people, many of whom are very much the kinds of questionable characters I'm naturally drawn to (Trump, Bill Cosby, O. J. Simpson, Imelda Marcos) – is what appears to be a deep sense of grievance and resentment on Ruby's part against me specifically for having (as she sees it) stolen her career. I'd heard through the grapevine over the years that she had a problem with me, resented me, viewed me as her enemy, and then more recently on an appearance on Adam

Buxton's podcast, when asked about me, she'd said that hearing my name made her want to vomit.

All of this, it was felt, would contribute to an awkwardness that would add piquancy to the interview, but I certainly didn't want to cancel at short notice and give her more of a reason to hate me.

I soldiered on. It's not the most physically demanding exercise, sitting at your desk and speaking to someone on a screen for a couple of hours. I had decided to open the conversation by clearing the air and the you-make-me-vomit comment and her feelings about me generally, her anger, her envy, whatever it was. She was, immediately, gracious and apologetic. She said she'd had a kind of fixation on the idea that I'd killed off her career, because I rose at a time her star was waning on TV, but it wasn't really *me*, she said. It was something I represented. She said she once had to leave a restaurant because she saw someone wearing a Louis Theroux T-shirt.

She talked about her mental health and about being institutionalized over the years. One episode was triggered by a home renovation when she was presented with a leaflet of paint colours that was so exhaustive and finely differentiated that the quantity of choices sent her into a spin – a pyschosis triggered by a Dulux colour chart. Another story involved a trip across America to promote a book about wellness or mindfulness or something similar during which she had a breakdown, which struck me as the possible premise of a film: the camera pans from the smiling photos of the author holding copies of her book full of mental health bromides to the sobbing crumpled heap of a human who can't leave her room.

I'd watched hours of her old shows in preparation and had transcribed sections. I'd been told by one of her long-time collaborators that she has a terrible memory and can't recall much about making her programmes, so I was able to rely on my notes to reconstruct some of the encounters. Her day with Trump – which

I remembered watching when it went out – took place in 1999 or thereabouts and came on the heels of one of his early flirtations with a presidential run. She boards his plane and they quickly don't click. 'Why do you want to be president?' she asks. 'Would you able to date?' It says something for his acuity that he sees her coming so early and so clearly. 'You're angry with a smile,' he says. Ruby gets into his limo without the camera but you can hear her on mike babbling and confessing her emotional frailties and seeming to seek his forgiveness.

Ruby was hard on her old programmes, reproaching herself for asking gauche questions, while I told her, honestly, that I thought her opening question – asking Trump about his dating – was a reasonable first salvo, cheeky but not offensive. What else was she going to ask him about, his economic policy? In a similar vein, she was self-lacerating about an interview she'd done with Madonna, though to be honest here too I thought she'd made a decent fist of the encounter, capturing the brittleness and control freakery of the legendary songstress – the key moment comes when Madonna tells off a cameraman because she thinks he has squashed an expensive suitcase.

In fact, I don't know if I mentioned this, it's her more famous ones that I find myself appreciating maybe less than I should – Imelda Marcos, Tammy Faye Baker – where Ruby is so firmly in control the encounters run the risk of being too easy. Imelda famously sang karaoke while Ruby made faces into the camera, whereas in the Cosby interview, he, like Trump, takes against her early on, and commences a semi-comical meta-commentary about her approach, picking up a prop phone receiver and announcing into it, 'She's still talking . . . It's sort of like listening to an answering machine you don't know how to fix.'

I told her I believed there was more mileage in her old footage for a revisit series, somewhat in the style of the one I'd done. She was more grateful for this than she had any need to be, and we finished the chat after two hours plus, the hatchet buried, at which point whatever illness I've been labouring under returned, and for the rest of the day I was semi-useless.

Friday 16 October

We are now in some new phase of the pandemic that involves, according to a recent government announcement, three tiers or levels of restriction on activity. No one can agree whether they go too far or not far enough, they just know that it's either one or the other. The virus is rampaging across the country. Hospitals aren't yet overrun so there is maybe a vague feeling of disbelief in the background . . . Will this really happen? Is it being overhyped? Whispers of a second lockdown. Some call it a 'circuit breaker', but the children are at school, so it isn't like before. The only change on that front is that we do Ray's drop-off while wearing masks, walking across the school grounds via designated one-way paths and then stopping behind a little metal rail.

Nights are an alternate rota between Nancy and me – one does Ray, the other one does the other two. Increasingly the older boys seem the more onerous responsibility since they resist being in bed before 11 p.m. and I just want to go up at 10.30. Jack then decides he wants to have a shower. Then read one of his manga comic books. At least there are fewer arguments between them now Arthur is permanently upstairs in the top room. They are less like a volatile and physically abusive couple.

Life goes on. This week we heard BBC Two wants to do our snooker idea – 'Ball Gods', renamed 'Snookered' or possibly 'Pocket Gods' or 'Snooker Gods'. And we push on with other ideas, including 'Tell Them You Love Me', a film about the relationship between an American academic and a profoundly disabled man – they were either a loving couple or a predator and her victim depending on who you believe. Nancy seems happier – maybe relieved is the word – that we are sprouting the green shoots of Mindhouse being a successful business. In a difficult time there are signs our production company is inching forward with commissions that don't involve me . . . and I am excited to get going and only slightly chagrined that I didn't maybe do it years earlier.

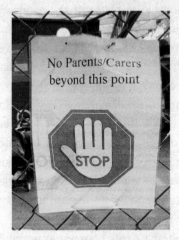

School protocol.

Sunday 18 October

On Saturday, Nancy had taken Ray to the park. I was at home doing laundry and tidying and organizing his toys, listening to a podcast about a missing Bulgarian con artist, the crypto-queen, when she called.

'He's fine,' she'd said, 'but Ray had a reaction to a brownie or maybe a cookie from the cafe and an ambulance came and we're at the hospital.'

The time had stretched on. Texts were coming in with updates, mainly to do with how boring it was and how long they were having to wait. It being a Saturday, I began thinking about having a drink and knew there was very little in the cabinet other than Cointreau and Aperol and bitters and two bottles of port. And some beer in the fridge. Around 5.30 I drove out to get some olive oil and came back with the olive oil plus a bottle of Gentleman Jack bourbon and some Hendricks gin.

'Big party tonight,' the Kurdish man had said, and for some reason gave me a free Ritter Sport, marzipan flavour, maybe to add to the fun. Gin rickeys, with Ritter Sport chasers.

Back at the house I'd realized there was no tonic so I made a gin cocktail out of old crystallized honey that I liquefied in the microwave and ice and fresh lime juice and soda water. It was delicious. I drank several more in fairly quick succession, while I'd peeled potatoes and par-boiled them and got the chicken on.

Nancy was sending more texts from the hospital. Her phone was about to die and could I arrange an Uber? The logic of me arranging an Uber for her if her phone wasn't working escaped me – how would I coordinate the pick-up?

Jump in a black cab, I texted. **Use your card.**

I haven't brought my card, she texted back.

Can't you borrow a charger or just buy one?

Buy one in kids a&e???!!!! And then: **Don't write stupid shit.**

By the time she and Ray got back I was listening to LSD – the supergroup involving Labrinth, Sia and Diplo – on the kitchen speaker and enjoying it maybe a little too much. *I'm a gee-gee-gee-gee-gee gee-gee-genius.* I made Nancy a cocktail and then made myself another one, then I drank both of them, since she was dawdling – you snooze you lose – then made two more, improvising a drink involving bourbon and lime juice.

With Ray, we watched an episode of *Dr Who* in which the doctor, played by David Tennant, went back to 1599 and met Shakespeare. The Globe was being used as a portal to another planet or another dimension by alien witch creatures. The Doctor kept saying things like 'Once more unto the breach' and Shakespeare would say 'That's good, I might use that.' I had a hunch I might be hammered, or on the verge of it, because I kept thinking how funny and well written the episode was. When it finished I took Ray up. It was too late for a story but he asked me to lie with him a minute.

'What did it feel like when you ate the cookie?' I asked.

'First my tongue was itchy,' he said. 'Then it felt like my throat was full of mud. Then my eyes were itchy.'

'It must have been scary,' I said.

'It was scary when I went in the amblience,' he said. 'Can you send Mummy up to give me a kiss?'

But after I left the room he was asleep within seconds.

Downstairs I took a Nurofen and had another drink and listened to the LSD album again on Spotify while tidying the kitchen and washing up.

Around four in the morning I awoke fully clothed on the sofa, my mouth dry with the weird feeling of having been doused in alcohol. I was weather-beaten, sodden, shipwrecked on the shores of Pisshead's Cove. I thought of all the booze in my body and I felt remorseful and told myself I should probably dump all the gin and bourbon down the sink. But it had cost nearly eighty pounds, and was I really the kind of person who can't keep spirits in the house? Did I drink too much? Was I struggling? Did I care?

At 7.30, Ray and I got up and came downstairs. I was feeling rough but mindful of the need to keep Ray amused and I spent forty-five minutes trying to download stories onto a device he has called a Lunii, a little box which tells bedtime stories to children. The app was infernal: to find the stories I had to download some software onto my laptop, and create an account. Then I had to find a charging cable when the first one didn't work . . . it was like a twenty-first-century fatherhood *Krypton Factor* being performed with a hangover and Ray peering over my shoulder, growing impatient.

'It should work now, no hang on . . .'

'I want to do something else,' he said.

'I think I've got it. Look.'

Then we started a puzzle, laying it out on the floor as I wondered how hungover I was. By 10 a.m. I felt relatively normal.

Nancy did her Peloton and I stumbled through a vicious Joe Wicks, 'Seven Days of Sweat 2020 Day 6' . . . which had no breaks between the exercises. I showered and listened to the LSD album on my phone in the bathroom. Nancy was outside and said, 'You're obsessed.'

'I just like the album. No biggie.'

Afterwards, downstairs, Nancy said: 'I need to talk to you.'

'Go on.'

'Tell me honestly. How drunk were you last night?'

'On a curry scale, I was madras-level drunk but not vindaloo drunk.'

'What is happening to you?' she said. 'You never used to be like this.'

'Well, it was a Saturday night so I decided to cut loose.'

'But it's not just on Saturday nights. What was your excuse last Monday night?'

'If you are saying I have been drinking too much I think you are probably correct,' I said, wondering at my use of the word 'probably'.

'You were in charge of the kids.'

'I was, but I think they were well taken care of.' I thought about the roast chicken and the potatoes. 'I wasn't smashed.'

'We don't spend any time together.'

'Well, we watched *Doctor Who* together.'

'For about ten minutes.'

'Half an hour. I can still remember most of what happened so I can't have been that drunk.'

'You're just not here. You're not present. You're in your bubble of alcohol. Going off to have bore-bons. You never used to do that.'

'It's pronounced berben. A bore-bon is a kind of biscuit.'

After lunch we went to Highgate Woods – me, Nancy, Art and Ray. As we walked along the path a woman in her fifties or sixties coming towards us looked at me as she passed and said, 'You are fantastic.'

'Ha ha! Thanks!'

'It's like a permanent ego boost,' I said to Nancy when she was gone. 'Random strangers telling you you're amazing. Everyone should have that.'

We headed deeper into the woods, past a grove with half-finished bivouacs put there by an aspirant Bear Grylls and fallen trees which Ray climbed and tried to walk along. We emerged onto a path where a whimsical-looking older man was sitting on a bench, next to a fancy old bicycle.

'Shame you didn't get Jimmy,' he said, with no preamble. I recognized it as a reference to Jimmy Savile, the DJ, charity fundraiser and prolific sex offender, who, depending on your point of view, I either made a revealing programme about or failed to make a revealing programme about.

'Ha! Can't win them all,' I said, thinking, *Here we go*, and without slowing down.

'I'm from Leeds. I knew him,' he said.

'Everyone from Leeds knew him, didn't they?'

I was past him now and moving fast. As I walked off, he said after me: '*He'll haunt you!*'

'So I guess it kind of evens out,' I said to Nancy afterwards. 'You're fantastic. You'll be haunted by Jimmy Savile.'

Friday 23 October

I had taken Ray to his swimming class after school, and then afterwards, on the way home, we stopped off at the park. In the playground a couple of older boys were on the big round swing. One might have been twelve or thirteen, the other a little younger. I thought about asking them to move along.

'Hey, guys, would it be OK if he went on the swing?'

'We're on it.'

'I know but . . . he's five and this is a playground for small children.'

'Says who?'

'Ha ha! Seriously, though, guys, I'm asking you as a favour, if you don't mind . . . Go on, it would mean a lot to the kid.'

'Make us.'

'Listen, guys, I'm trying to be nice. Now just fuck off before this turns nasty.'

None of this conversation took place. We just waited, and then eventually another swing came free, a non-round one, and I pushed Ray for ten minutes or so on that.

'I want the highest number, Daddy . . .'

I thought about all the times I'd pushed swings, going back to Arthur thirteen or more years ago. I felt I'd spent a lifetime pushing children on swings and, God forgive me, I thought, *I've had enough of this*, and I found some of my resentment and frustrations boiling over into OVER-pushing, pushing the swing so hard it went high enough that the chains slackened and the seat shook and there seemed a possibility of Ray falling off . . . Ray naturally loved it, gasped and laughed with excitement.

Then the big swing came free. I pushed Ray on that.

'Not from the back, from the front,' Ray said.

He wanted me to say, 'Mummy won't believe you!' which was something I chanted once before, five or six months ago, when he'd dropped an ice cream on a swing and he'd wanted to blame it on me. *Mummy won't believe you!* It had made him laugh. This time, I pushed and pushed, higher and higher, as his head lay on the back of the round metal ring, bouncing as he swung up and down, and I remembered a time in Harlesden, at Roundwood Park, when I'd put in a similar level of effort with Jack, pushing and pushing, on the edge of frenzy and frustration, making a deal with myself to give him every bit of swing-based excitement he could imagine, not to call time on it until *he* said he'd had enough, and we'd arrived home and Jack said he had a headache and then vomited, and this time with Ray I became conscious of not putting too much stress on his head, and not bouncing his brain too much.

'We do need to go home, Ray, Mummy's expecting us.'

We rode home – him on his scooter and me on my bike – he scooted the whole way on his own, and we arrived back at 5.30 or so.

'I don't want to go on the iPad,' Ray said. 'I want to do a activity. Can we do Consequences?'

He was talking about the drawing game: you do a silly head, fold it over, swap it around, do a torso, fold it over, and so on. There was a nano-pause – of surprise and confusion as my mind short-circuited over the possibility of saying, *No you can't do an activity you have to go on the iPad*, before I said, 'Great idea, let's do Consequences' and we played a couple of rounds. Then I put some pre-fab pizza in the oven and he went on the iPad.

Saturday 24 October

The second proto-semi-lockdown is so boring that I can't find it in me to write about it. I don't know what supposed tier we are at in London; maybe two? I do know that Wales is in lockdown as of today. Infection rates climbing across Europe. People dying at a slower rate due, apparently, to more knowledge of the virus and its ways. The news is a litany of Covid updates. Andy Burnham, Mayor of Greater Manchester, in the news for demanding fully costed aid from central government, which they have refused.

Thursday night was the latest and last presidential debate . . . The main change since the last one being the installation of mute buttons to stop candidates talking over each other. Trump boasting that a Covid vaccine would be ready in weeks and that thanks to various drugs he'd been taking he was now 'immune' to the disease. Biden pointing out that 220,000 Americans have died. 'People are learning to live with it,' Trump said. 'People are learning to live with it?' Biden came back. 'People are learning to die with it.'

On the radio, as I made lunch, on *Any Answers*, a man was saying: 'I think the younger people are having to pay the price for the unwillingness of older people to take the necessary risks. Even if some older people do die, life needs to continue.'

The host asked the man his age. 'Seventy-eight,' he said.

'Are you saying some lives are worth more than others?'

Man: 'I think I am.'

Wednesday 28 October

Losehill Park Hotel, Hope, Derbyshire

For the last four nights we have been ensconced in a smart hotel in the Peak District, having driven up from London. Feels almost surreal being catered to in such high style – tables with white linen, bright breakfast room with choices of pastries and fresh juices and everyone talking in hushed voices, as light streams through the high windows. After so many years of Airbnbs, to stay in an actual hotel where they clean your room and make your meals is revelatory. For the first couple of days the kids were in awe of the level of treatment, behaving as though they'd been transported into Downton Abbey on a probationary basis, reprimanding each other if they spotted what they thought was a lapse in decorum.

'Jack, that's the wrong knife. You're supposed to be using a butter knife.'

'Arthur's waffling so hard about cutlery. He thinks he's a cutlery OG.'

On our first day we drove to a visitors' centre on the edge of Buxton and bundled out into blustering rain and wind, maps flapping, inadequately apparelled in puffer jackets (the boys) that soaked up rain and a vast tentlike purple cagoule (me) that wasn't in fact anywhere close to waterproof. My gloves were water magnets, my purple freaking cagoule was a joke, my only trump card was my Blundstone boots, bought for me by Nancy for Christmas last year. We made our way up through the woods and were dry for a while. The boys went off-piste and were exploring and jumping off logs and finding side interests . . . berms and fallen trees and undergrowth.

It was a pleasant surprise to find that the old childhood pursuits still held some appeal. I remembered being young and walking up hills in the Dorset countryside around Beaminster, with names like Lewesden and Pilsden Pen.

At the bottom, wearing masks, we bought hot chocolates for the kids and a Peak District colouring book for Ray, then sat in a marquee and sipped our drinks. I googled local outdoor gear stores and after we'd finished our refreshments we went down the pedestrianized high street and spent an hour buying new hats and jackets and gloves and waterproof trousers, then went back to the hotel to jump in the indoor pool. Nancy told Ray not to dive down into the hot tub because his hair might get caught in the pump and he'd drown. Arthur said he'd seen an episode of *Curious and Unusual Deaths* that related a similar case of a girl getting stuck to the bottom of a swimming pool. After that, Ray, not surprisingly, refused to go back into the hot tub.

In the evening they put us in a small private dining room that adjoined the main restaurant, the five of us in our own little area – it was hard to tell whether this was a promotion, on the grounds that we were esteemed guests, or a relegation due to us being seen as a problem family. The private nature of our nook gave it an atmosphere of aristocratic grandeur, which briefly had a civilizing effect on Arthur and Jack. Alas, it was short-lived.

'Riots in Philadelphia,' Nancy said. 'Police killed a black man called Walter Wallace.'

'That's why BLM is important,' Arthur said.

'Arthur thinks he's a BLM boss,' Jack said.

'Jack is turning alt-right,' Arthur said.

'You're waffling so hard right now,' Jack said.

'He is. He's part of a TikTok group called "The Boys".'

'Just stop.'

I tried to play peace broker. 'Legitimate protest is important but looting isn't the answer.'

'No one said anything about looting,' Nancy said.

'Jack, where are you getting your information from?' I asked.

'YouTube. Sorry, but rioting is just burning up other people's stuff. Not gonna lie.'

'Jack,' Arthur said. 'You have no idea.'

'Arthur you are such a simp. You literally like anything about sexual assault. "I am scared because there is a man walking behind me."'

'What are you on about, Jack?' I asked.

'There is a selfie from a woman and there's a man literally minding his own business walking behind her and she says, "If I die tonight then this man did it."'

'Oh.'

'It's all over TikTok, people just trying to get more followers by liking random stuff about sexual assault.'

I said to Nancy, 'We've got the Balkanization of the Internet made flesh right here.'

Ray, meanwhile, was eating bread and doing some colouring.

On subsequent days we visited Chatsworth, the stately home – the house itself was closed but the grounds were open – and Peveril Castle, and a warren of limestone caverns which had once been home to a community of rope makers, whose ropes had been used for the mining of lead in the late eighteenth century.

Today was Ray's birthday. He is six. We'd brought the presents with us in the car – a new marble run from Granny, some magic marker pens, colouring books, activity books, some Lego, an Usborne superhero sticker book. The sticker book characters are not licensed from an existing comic franchise. They have been invented by Usborne and have names like Voide and Vulkano.

Jack said to Ray: 'Ray, which superhero universe do you prefer, Marvel or Usborne?'

Ray wasn't sure how to answer this though he seemed to suspect he was being satirized.

'Ray! Ray! Which is your favourite Usborne superhero? My favourite is Mega-Prawn! He is so awesome!'

'Jack!' Nancy said.

'Mega-Prawn isn't an Usborne superhero, Jack,' I said. 'Stop being silly.'

'Ray, who do you think would win in a fight between Mega-Prawn and Iron Man?'

'Jack!'

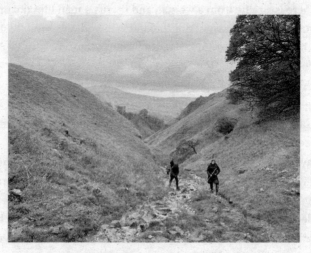

Peak District landscape with rambling family.

Friday 30 October

We drove back to London yesterday. France and Germany are in lockdown now. US cases surpass 9 million 'with no end in sight', so says the *New York Times*, though death rates are down relative to infections. There were 280 deaths in the UK yesterday. And if that weren't enough there was a terrorist attack in France, another one (after a teacher being beheaded last week). This time three people were killed in a church in Nice. Apparently Macron had said something along the lines of 'we will keep doing cartoons' which was received in some Muslim communities not as 'we will exercise free speech' but as 'we will keep doing cartoons of Muhammad.'

Last night we were out with two other couples at a restaurant in Soho for Musician Friend's birthday. We drank cocktails and ate at a table out on the pavement, while a trickle of homeless people came up and asked for money and a smaller trickle of drunken passers-by asked for selfies.

'Sorry, I don't carry money,' I said, truthfully.

'But what do you do if you're homeless now that no one carries cash? How are you supposed to get money?' Nancy said.

'In the future they'll have devices,' Musician Friend said. 'It's Elon Musk and the cyborgs. He says we're already cyborgs. We'll have chips and wave them at your phone. Or maybe you'll plant your thumb on their phone . . .'

'I'm getting the mince and potatoes,' Actor Friend said. 'Apparently it was Jimmy Savile's favourite dish.'

'That would make sense, his teeth were so bad, he didn't like food that was hard to chew,' I said.

A little later a drunk man came up with two or three *Big Issue*s in one hand and said, 'Spare a few quid? It would be greatly appreciated at this difficult time.'

'No money, sorry mate.'

'None of us has cash.'

'I take cards.'

I thought it was a joke but then from the pockets of his coat he brought out a phone and a chip-and-pin device. He punched in three pounds and I held my card against his machine. After it went through, he said, 'You don't want this piece of shit, do you?'

'Yes, I do,' I said.

On the way back home, on the train, I read the *Big Issue*'s interviews with Eddie Hearn the sports manager and electronic music pioneer Gary Numan, and thought, *It's a little thin but I wouldn't call it 'shit'.*

Saturday 31 October

Halloween. And the monster bringing bone-chills and nightmares to the globe is a nano-scopic virus called Covid-19. Even I am getting tired of recruiting pandemic into metaphors.

News comes that a second lockdown is on its way. Total number seriously ill in hospital in the UK with Covid is 10,000, accounting for fewer than 10 per cent of NHS beds, but the numbers are allegedly doubling every something days. The situation is outpacing the worst predictions of a few weeks ago, they say. It's strange because, when you don't know many or any people who are seriously ill, it feels faintly unreal.

Joe Wicks did a Halloween Special workout wearing a costume, with family also costumed. I did it later in the day. He announced there were 6,000 or maybe 7,000 viewers live on the live stream, saying it full of excitement, despite him once having nearly a million people tuning in.

We are back where we were.

November 2020

I SHOT JOE EXOTIC

Wednesday 4 November

In the middle of the night Nancy woke me, sounding upset, saying, 'Trump's won again.'

'No, seriously?' I said.

We had had a bad night. Jack had had a disturbed sleep and it was 2 or 3 a.m. before I'd drifted off. At 7.45 my alarm went off and I went down with Ray and made tea. We played with Lego while I tried to listen to the election and do all the usual kitchen duties of unloading the dishwasher while Nancy wrangled the older kids. As more reports came in, it became clear the election was, in fact, still in the balance. Florida had gone to Trump, the big one – if Biden had won it that would have been game over – but both candidates still had a path. Massive doubt and anxiety on the Democrat side. Texas had gone for Trump too, and Ohio, but Arizona was leaning Biden and Georgia was too close to call. Likewise Nevada, and more and more it looked like the traditionally blue states that had swung Trump in 2016 would decide the election again – Michigan, Wisconsin, Pennsylvania.

I took Ray to school, following the new one-way route, via the infants' entrance, only to discover I had forgotten my mask, and also, as it turned out, the Usborne *Amazing Maze Pirate Activity Book* I was supposed to bring.

'I'll drop it off at the school office,' I said.

'No, it's NOT FOR SCHOOL,' Ray said.

'OK, it's for after school? I'll drop it round with Sophia.' (His childminder.)

Ray was still not moving.

'Ray-ray, we need to get a move on or we'll be late.'

'Mmgh!'

'Come on, little guy. We're going to get in trouble.'

After some more wheedling from me, he gave in and sloped into class. I walked back to collect my bike, passing the Catering Dad who sold me pasta at the beginning of Lockdown One.

'How you doing?' he said.

'Yeah, OK. You?'

'Groundhog Day,' he said, not, ironically enough, for the first time.

Back at home I gathered up my things – backpack, headphones, bike keys.

'Where are you going?' Nancy said.

'I'm getting a blood test. And then I'm going to get my hair cut.'

The blood test was so I can go on the Joe Exotic shoot. It had been booked in at a clinic on Harley Street, on the top floor of one of those large Regency houses. I ascended the wide staircase, feeling a little like I was seeing a tutor at Oxford, the age and grandeur of the building brought a sense of performance. After a twenty-minute wait, the doctor came out, a younger Eastern European or possibly Russian woman, wearing a mask.

'Blood test,' I said. 'For antibodies.'

'Are you going anywhere?'

'I might be travelling for work.'

'Little scratch.'

Later I thought about the phrase 'little scratch' and wondered if it might be a way of avoiding the phallic connotations of 'little prick'.

'So what do you make of all of this?' the doctor asked.

'The whole situation?'

'Yes,' she said.

'I'm mainly confused. I guess I can't work out if we're locked down too much or not enough. I'm not sure. What do you think?'

'Completely between us?' she asked.

'Of course.'

'I thought the system of local lockdown was doing the job. Look, the reality is, Covid is going to be with us a long, long time. And we have to learn to live with it. The damage to the economy, the people out of work, I can't say it's worth it. We know why the second surge happened. Students going off to university. But the truth is, not a single student has even died from Covid. We know so much more now than we did in the spring. We know how to care for people. I do understand why they thought they had to do it but it's not going to make much difference at the end of the day.'

She talked about patients she had in private practice with advanced cervical cancer who had gone untreated in the NHS due to Covid.

'GPs are afraid to see patients,' she said.

'Wait, they're afraid to see patients? Or patients are afraid to see them?'

'GPs are afraid because they don't have social distancing measures in their waiting rooms. Do you know the average age of people dying with Covid?'

'Between late seventies and early eighties?'

'The measures have a place, but they can't be considered in isolation. We need also to think about some metric that factors in quality of life. Risk reduction for someone in their eighties also has consequences for the physical and mental health of someone in their teens.'

Afterwards, I killed time at Pret A Manger making calls and sending emails and sipping coffee with my sweaty mask around my neck, while I waited to see Karen, my hairdresser, who I hadn't visited for more than six months. She's cut my hair for fifteen years or more, and been an informal sounding board and low-key therapeutic presence in my life, and I'd thought about her in the early months of the pandemic, wondering how she was getting on, but with so much still unsettled and more measures looming it was unlikely to be the joyful reunion we might have wished for. She'd been furloughed at home, she told me. Asked how she'd been doing in general, she said, 'Ghastly.'

I cycled home listening to a podcast about paedophiles, jumped on a Zoom call, dropped off Ray's maze book with Sophia, then did a quick Joe Wicks. By now they were saying Biden had won Wisconsin and had maybe edged ahead. The alt-right on Twitter all claiming the fix was in, lefties saying maybe Biden had a chance. Trump demanding a recount in Wisconsin.

Nancy and I had planned to have a last night out but also a new tumble dryer was being delivered – the old one that came with the house has finally given up the ghost – so we ordered sushi and with the big boys we watched the last episode of a German series on Netflix called *Barbarians*. It follows the lead-up to the legendary Battle of Teutoburg Forest, where three Roman legions were decimated by the local tribes, after being betrayed by an inside man. It was all in German and Latin with subtitles, expensive and a little silly and landing squarely in the sweet spot of a family looking for a middle ground between their young teenagers looking for satisfying action and an old guard grateful for anything vaguely informative and historical.

As I write this, a *New York Times* alert has come in saying: 'Biden's path to victory grows.'

Last day before new lockdown kicks in tomorrow.

Thursday 5 November

A polite but no less scary legal letter has come in from lawyers acting for the *Tiger King* production. It apparently prohibits us from having any further contact with a number of contributors we have been lining up for our Joe Exotic visit, including (but not limited to) John Reinke, John Finlay, Tim Stark, Eric Love (who leads 'Team Tiger', the outfit trying to get Joe pardoned), and Joe himself. I forwarded it on to Arron with a message, 'Have you seen this?' and an exploding head emoji.

If we go ahead and have any further contact we will be liable for 'tortious interference'. I have no idea what this even means. But it could be very expensive, I'm told – to the tune of hundreds of thousands. As it stands, we are supposedly not even allowed to let the people we are in touch with know that we can't have any further contact with them. However there's nothing in the letter about the Baskins, Joe's lawyer Francisco, and one or two other friends and relations. 'It doesn't blow us out of the water . . . but we have to proceed carefully,' I wrote.

Reading all the legal verbiage got my dander up. We will have to respond through our lawyers. Arron spoke to one of them and then called back. 'He thinks we're still OK to use all the material from our rushes.'

'Well, Jesus, I never imagined we might *not* be OK to use that stuff. We shot it in 2011!'

'I'm just letting you know what he said,' Arron replied.

Friday 6 November

Did two consecutive corporates, one at 2 p.m. for treasurers groups in which I couldn't nail the concept of what a treasurer was.

'Thanks for all your hard work totting up numbers,' I said at the end.

'That was great, except one tiny thing,' the client said. 'Treasurers don't really tot up numbers, that's more accountants.'

'OK, no problem, I'll do it again.' We went again, dropping in for my goodbye. 'And *thanks for all your hard work bringing in the money!*'

'OK . . . ah . . . great.'

'Did I get it wrong?'

'No, you're . . . fine.'

The event had been advertised as a free-form conversation, with anecdotes from the road and observations about the human condition. It isn't going out until next week but they wanted some comments about the election and Trump, and they were keen for it not to feel too dated, meaning I really needed to talk as though the results are now in. 'Fine,' I said. 'I think it's pretty clear he's lost.' And in the exchange that followed I confidently spoke about his defeat in the past tense, even though it hadn't happened, and almost immediately afterwards felt a kind of quiet panic set in, that this was an unnecessary high-risk strategy on my part, announcing speculative future events as firm facts, and that it might end up being my 'Dewey Defeats Truman' moment.

At 4 p.m. I had another event booked, a podcast for a mysterious US company based in San Francisco that specializes in CRM, which I googled and discovered means 'customer relationship management', often using 'cloud-based solutions' to 'optimize outcomes'. OK then! Wholly out of my depth on the tech side, I talked instead about relationships and connection – which is after all what I specialize in, I suppose – and the necessity of recognizing that we're all struggling and focusing on the closeness that can result when we are honest about how hard it is. I closed with a quote from the Hungarian Holocaust survivor and Nobel Prize-winning author Imre Kertész, whose wise and searingly honest books, quite truthfully, I've never read (that was one of my jokes), but who once said in an interview in *Newsweek*: 'I experienced my most radical moments of happiness in the concentration camp. You cannot imagine what it's like to be allowed to lie in the camp's hospital, or to have a ten-minute break from indescribable labour. To be very close to death is also a kind of happiness. Just surviving becomes the greatest freedom of all.'

Saturday 7 November

In the morning my low-level freak-out at having confidently announced a Biden victory as though it had already happened at the corporate event for the mysterious treasurers began to escalate. It seemed likely that even next week the race might still be undecided. Would the video be leaked on the Internet, and what would that mean for me – trusted BBC information source and lockdown Vera Lynn, caught purveying fiction as fact? I emailed my agent to let her know the situation. 'Please can you let them know they might need to nip that bit out.' Then, late afternoon, news came: Biden had enough votes from Pennsylvania. CNN called it first. Other outlets followed in quick succession and my Twitter feed was a torrent of triumphalism, 'You're fired!' 'Bye-bye, Orange Man.' 'We should extend the olive branch of reconciliation right after we finish gloating.' 'Fuck off you bigoted twat.' And so on.

Trumpers were talking about alleged errors and irregularities and promising to pursue legal challenges. No concession speech from Trump, likewise no concession from congressional leaders.

The sense of relief is undercut by awareness that Trump would undoubtedly have won had it not been for the virus. Also, big Trump gains among almost every non-white demographic and major Trump support among Hispanic people in Miami-Dade. Still it was a respite from the cascade of depressing lockdown news – corona cases surging, three successive days of more than 100,000 new cases in the US, and one day with more than 1,000 deaths.

Sunday 8 November

On Radio 4 they ran an interview David Frost had done with Biden in 1987, when he was making his first presidential run. Biden was cogent and considered and thoughtful, talking about the need for equal opportunity and social justice.

'I'd vote for this guy,' Nancy said. 'What happened to him?'

'He got old,' I said.

'Why did he lose?'

'Got into trouble for plagiarizing a speech by Neil Kinnock.'

A few minutes later Biden was actually saying, 'I've been following the UK election and something the Labour candidate, Neil Kinnock, said, really hit home with me. He said, why am I the first one in my family who went to university? Why is my wife the first in her family to go to university? Were my forefathers all thick? Were they not hard working enough – these men who went down the pit, worked a full day, then went and played football for two hours? Or did they not have a platform to achieve?'

'That's the bit he plagiarized,' I said. 'How funny.'

At eleven, we turned in. I lay on my side reading a longish article about the election and Trumpism and where it goes now. Nancy was reading something on her phone. She rolled over and said: 'We don't know each other anymore.'

'You're so busy,' I said.

'Stop it.'

'You've got your hands full with work,' I said. 'Starting Mind-house.' This was facetious but also not.

'We need to book another break.'

'At a hotel.'

'But who will look after the kids?'

I was thinking, *Arthur?* But could we leave him in charge of Jack for that long?

'I don't know,' I said. 'We need to reconnect.'

We kissed. I wondered if intimacy might be on the cards.

'I need to brush my teeth,' I said. When I came back, she had her sleep mask on and her light was out.

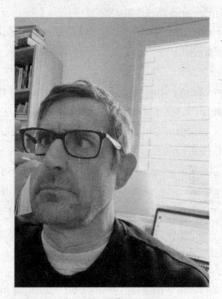

Insert and rotate.

Monday 9 November

Tampa, Florida

First trip back to the States in more than a year.

It felt sad leaving the house. More so than it used to pre-Covid. I felt like I was abandoning the site of a plane crash, leaving the few survivors to fend for themselves while I went to seek help. My position was perilous but I had the advantage of taking positive action. Their task was simply to survive.

The last couple of days had been a crescendo of anxiety and hypomania on my part and tension coming from Nancy. Each night, I'd put Ray down and then tidy the kitchen, trying to put in some good deeds to offset my going away.

Trump still not conceding defeat. Which in a way is not surprising, since isn't that his brand? And isn't that what those who love him love him for? Violating norms and refusing to observe the conventions of fair play?

I'd been up since 7 a.m. with Ray and used leftover batter to make pancakes. I brewed coffee and got Ray dressed.

'You're all happy,' Nancy said.

'I'm not all happy. I feel weird leaving you alone with the kids.'

I took Ray off to school. I was on the bike and he was on the scooter. It was warm for late autumn and dry and the streets were quiet. No gloves or hats needed. He sped along and we got there fast. Parents and children were milling at the gates. In the small playground outside the door to his classroom he said, 'I want to give you a big hug.'

'Let me get down on your level,' I said and kneeled.

'I don't want you to go to America, Daddy.'

'I know, but I'll make sure I call and we can speak on video.'

He turned and went in without complaint, which was maybe

the most heartbreaking part of it, that and looking at his back as he went in, with his cheap nylon satchel and his water bottle. He stood in the doorway talking to a friend – I wondered if he might look back at me and I lingered in case he did, then he smiled at his friend, and I could see he was in his own world now. I walked back to my bike.

I went to the chemist to get some masks, then went home and packed, and at a little after ten I climbed into my taxi.

My producer, director and sound recordist all flew yesterday, using visa waivers and work exemptions to get through. I was allowed to fly because it's for work and I have a US passport. The airport – Heathrow Terminal 5 – was empty. Some seats were taped off, restaurants closed, everyone in masks. The flight had barely anyone on it.

On the plane I drank a Bloody Mary and then, with the meal, one of those little bottles of Cabernet Sauvignon. I had another, and then two more, possibly three. I was catching up on research, listening to a multi-part podcast about Joe. Feeling the effect of the wine, I kept taking off my glasses to write notes on my iPhone, since I can see better up-close without them, then losing the glasses. At one point I was despairing of ever finding them again. I hadn't brought a spare pair and I had a feeling of mounting panic as I looked under my chair, in the seat pockets, in the toilets and still couldn't find them. Then I touched the top of my head. There they were. Relief mixed with shame and chagrin.

At Miami airport several long slow-moving queues snaked around the area in front of the immigration desks. Bleary and jet-lagged, I scrolled through Twitter and the *New York Times* on my phone. Trump and the Republicans still not conceding. A crazy Trump lawyer, a woman called Sidney Powell, was circulating conspiracy theories to do with the election and vote rigging and

Venezuela, so outlandish in content that even Tucker Carlson on Fox News had felt the need to distance himself from them.

I checked the feeds of the most rabid Trumpers. Scott Adams, the Dilbert cartoonist turned Trump acolyte, came across like a wrinkly necked American version of Comical Ali, the deranged PR guy who kept announcing that Saddam Hussein had won the Iraq War. Rumours were swirling of an event in DC this Saturday, some kind of right-wing anti-election protest. Disgusted right-wingers spitting chips over Fox News calling Arizona for Biden.

Lefties unsure whether we were in the midst of a Trump coup or just a political reality show staged on social media for the entertainment of his base. Jokes about the unintended comedy of the Giuliani press conference – announcing that the president would not concede at the Four Seasons Total Landscaping company in Philadelphia, between a crematorium and a sex shop. Evidently they thought they had booked the Four Seasons hotel. Hysteria on the news shows. Reports that Trump is installing 'loyalists' at the Pentagon. Biden planning his administration but almost all GOP lawmakers refusing to acknowledge he won the election and alleging large-scale fraud.

When I finally reached the immigration desk, I waved my US passport and the officer didn't even ask me any questions or take my temperature, simply saying: 'Mask and glasses off please.' And that was it. It was 8 p.m. when I got out, finding my driver from the car service. 'This way, Mr T', he said. Outside the air was hot and sticky though it was dark. For some reason, it was only now I thought about the fact there would be a four-and-a-half-hour drive to Tampa. En route, Jack the director called. We talked through the story.

'Seven thirty start,' Jack said.

I figured I'd be getting in past midnight. Six hours sleep if I was lucky. 'Why so early?'

'They are feeding the cats at 7.30 so it's our best chance of getting some action.'

The A/C was blasting against my leg. I pulled a hooded raincoat tight round me and tried to sleep.

Strange to be on my first trip back to America, in Florida, where Hurricane Eta bearing down on the state is the least of our worries. Yesterday there were 160,000 new Covid cases in the US. The US map of infections is blood-red down the middle, dripping from Illinois, Michigan, Indiana . . . the edges less bad. Graphs across the US and Europe show an upward ski jump of infections.

Friday 13 November

Four days in, and it's surreal how normal it feels to be away. The differences, having got here, are superficial: it's regular life, just with masks in the lobby, and hand gel everywhere, plastic cutlery in cellophane packets at breakfast, and the omelette cook sequestered behind a Perspex screen.

Day one, we met Carole and Howard Baskin – Carole being, of course, Joe's supposed nemesis and the target of his two murder-for-hire attempts. We toured Big Cat Rescue, the sanctuary where they house tigers rescued from tiger-breeding mills and roadside zoos, and where they strategize how to end tiger breeding in captivity, and also where Carole was, according to one of Joe's plots, supposed to be killed, by a felon on a bike path wielding a crossbow. She is polite, a little otherworldly, late fifties but with the air of a flower child in leopard-print attire. Howard is stooped, friendly, prone to crack corny jokes and make reference to my back catalogue, asking whether I thought he might have what it takes to be a rapper. The one moment of unexpectedly awkward comedy was a light-hearted bit of banter where I commented, without thinking, apropos of Carole, 'They do say the female of the species is deadlier than the male.' 'Definitely true in her case,' Howard joked, and then, realizing such dark humour would not play well given the accusations that Carole had killed a previous husband, looked pained. 'Please don't use that,' he said.

There is no avoiding the retrospective nature of the story. The action has largely happened, so much of what we filmed was a long conversation in a kitchen in the offices of Big Cat Rescue, as Howard and Carole, under my questioning, and appropriately Covid-distanced, recounted the story of how they'd first become aware of Joe Exotic, how they'd campaigned against him, and how they'd found out he was trying to have Carole killed.

The most powerful moment came when they played me a sampling of the voice messages they received in the wake of *Tiger King* airing. A deluge of misogynistic threats and abuse from anonymous trolls who had watched the series and decided that Carole was the true villain of the piece and felt the need to put her in further fear of her life. *'You fucked Joe. Now we're going to fuck you.' 'I'm going to put a bullet between your fuckin' eyes.' 'Just gettin' started, bitch. Just gettin' started.'*

From Tampa, we flew to Wichita, Kansas, via Chicago, staying just ahead of Hurricane Eta, filming a scene at the house of a couple of friends of Joe's who I'd met in 2011 – who were kind enough to cook me a steak, but alas didn't have much to offer in the way of revelation – and then on to Pauls Valley, Oklahoma, where we'd be staying. The drive was three and a half hours, straight down the middle of America. We'd started out at 6.30 a.m., passing water towers, wind turbines, grain elevators, wide vistas across flat open farmland.

In the afternoon we filmed with a niece of Joe's, Chealsi Putnam, a disgruntled former volunteer at Joe's zoo. She's in her early thirties and lives in the quiet rural house that belonged to Joe's parents. She has all the photos and memorabilia kept by Joe's mother; scrapbooks, DVDs of Joe's music career ('I Saw a Tiger', 'Starstruck') . . . She gave me three of Joe's DVDs, which have him on the cover looking airbrushed to the point of being plastinated, earrings, cowboy hat, blond mullet all present.

At the hotel, a Hampton Inn, Cath the producer said, 'We've booked you under the name Lewis Thomas. Just to be safe, in case word spreads that we're here.'

'Cool, like it. Never done that before. Like Paul McCartney. He used to travel as Paul Ramone I think.'

The woman at the front desk, who was heavyset, said: 'Name.'

'Lewis Thomas,' I said.

'ID please.'

'OK.' Pause to regroup. 'So for some reason they booked me in under the wrong name. My name is actually Louis Theroux.'

She took my licence. 'So why did they book you in as Lewis Thomas?'

'I don't know. I think they thought it was funny.' Then with what was intended as playful irony I said, 'Don't worry, heads will roll.'

She changed the name on the booking then looked up. I realized I was holding my three Joe Exotic DVDs against my chest. Her eyes went *zoop* down and then *zoop* back up again, while her expression didn't change.

'I'm Chrissie and this is Christie. If you need anything ya'll just holler.'

The pandemic is going extra-loco, 160,000 new cases, a million in ten days. Trump still hasn't conceded – naturally – and a far-right populist force of mainly conspiracy theorists, followers of Alex Jones, and far-right America First nationalists of the type we were supposed to be making a film about back in March is descending on Washington DC. Some cracks in the Republican ranks, a handful beginning to accept he's lost. Peak insanity arrived when, a few days after the debacle of the Four Seasons Landscaping press conference, Giuliani made another high-profile appearance to debunk the results of the election and appeared to start melting, like a malfunctioning robot, with black ink trickling from the area above his ears and down the side of his face.

The good news is, Nancy seems happier on calls. On Friday, Sophie calculated that with my commissions and other projects, we already have enough business coming through Mindhouse to keep going until next November.

In the evening we ate at a BBQ joint in Pauls Valley, a place I'd been to before called Bob's Pig Shop. On the walls were photos of men and women in galoshes with their hands jammed down the throats of catfish, blood trickling down their arms, though whether it's human blood or catfish blood isn't clear, maybe both? It's a practice called 'catfish noodling' – it involves pushing your fingers into the fish like a muff and flipping it out of the water. Pauls Valley is the catfish noodling capital of the world. Later it struck me, with the catfish blood and the human blood intermixing, noodling seems ideal for incubating new viral variants.

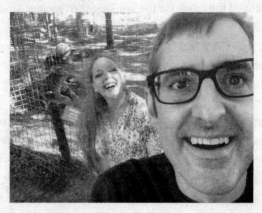

With Carole Baskin at Big Cat Rescue in Tampa, Florida.

Late November, exact date unknown

Some hotel in Oklahoma

I've done two weeks here in America. It seems a blur. Florida, to Kansas, to Oklahoma, to Texas. A safari of Joe Exotic's ex-colleagues, ex-friends, family members, enemies and survivors.

Each day felt like a surprise bonus moment of serendipity. After the strong start of Carole and Howard and then Chealsi, we drove down to Fort Worth, Texas, to meet Joe's disarmingly friendly lawyer, Francisco Hernandez, who, for reasons I can't quite fathom, though possibly due to the publicity it generates, is heavily involved in the quixotic campaign to have Joe pardoned. Francisco's office is a repository of Joe merch – devotional candles and paintings – and also a storage place for boxes containing the thousands of letters that come in from fans. 'He answers every single one,' said Francisco. And then, with pride, 'He is the most popular inmate in the history of America.' Strangely, he may not be far from the truth.

A few hours down the road, still in Texas, in a new-built evangelical church, we met with an old illusionist friend of Joe's, stage name Johnny Magic, who showed videos of them together in 2003 frolicking in a meadow with a young tiger and performing fundraisers for animals – Joe's presentational skills were charmingly inept. Then we drove to the far eastern border of the state, on the edge of Louisiana, for a sit-down with Joe's older brother Yarri, who's never spoken about Joe on TV before, and finally back to Joe's old park with Howard and Carole, who have taken possession of it, or what remains of it: an abandoned and dilapidated carcass, a graveyard and an ossuary, with fences pulled down, rubbish strewn around, obscene anti-Carole graffiti scrawled everywhere. 'EVIL BITCH.' 'DOOM ON YOU CUNT.'

Joe's old house, where he hosted us in 2011, and where I'd bottle-fed a baby tiger, was a ruin, the roof half caved in, with insulation and debris piled inside, old files and photos tipped out, letters, gay porn magazines, VHS tapes, ornaments and toys strewn amid animal excrement.

As the days passed, the picture of a vulnerable and unpredictable zookeeper came into sharper focus. Someone as charming as he was unscrupulous, who – as one of his friends put it – couldn't be alone, and who – in his brother Yarri's view – was like a cult leader, using his charm to manipulate those around him for money. He was pathologically dependent on love and companionship, and it was partly his need for lovers that had driven his financial chicanery: he'd taken donations for animals that were dead or had moved on, he'd used zoo funds to pay for quad bikes for his boyfriends, growing ever more blasé about the neglect of his animals.

Some of this ground had been covered in *Tiger King* but I also had the sense the series had underplayed aspects of Joe's unscrupulousness, and that for many viewers the distinction between what he had done – breeding and abusing animals – with what Carole did – saving animals and *not* breeding – had never completely punched through. The series had, unavoidably, ended up amplifying Joe's considerable charisma, and been a platform for his growing celebrity power, while also showing a Carole who, through no fault of her own, came across as unemotional, who perhaps gave off a sense of piety or judgement that viewers didn't warm to. In an odd way, it was all reminiscent of the face-off between Trump and Hillary Clinton – the primal id and the disapproving superego – and viewers couldn't help falling for Donald Exotic.

And so alongside the picture of Joe there grew in me a sense of annoyance at the *Tiger King* team and their legal intervention. 'They're very aggressive,' several contributors said. In my more embittered moments, spinning off into a kind of fever of self-righteousnesses, I perceived them as the apex predators in the ecosystem of the *Tiger King* phenomenon: the invisible antagonists, the most powerful and the wiliest figures in the entire drama, and I complained about them in scenes in my documentary, and I began thinking of ways to face them down while at the same time aware that what I was really doing was reacting out of my own self-interest and chastising them for actions not so different from things I'd done over the years.

Probably the most eye-opening moment in the last ten days – because of what it said about *me* – came late one evening at our hotel when Jack, my director, filmed me watching a clip from the outtakes of the 2011 documentary. It was my last ever interview with Joe. Joe had been elusive in the previous few days, but he'd agreed to come out for a final encounter, then quickly grew tired of my questions. 'This has all gone animal rights again,' he said, then lost his temper, and ripped off his mike. 'Yes, my animals are happy. No, I'm not going to stop breeding . . . Fuck you, fuck PETA, fuck Carole Baskin.' This outburst was memorably explosive, but what was more striking was what happened afterwards, which I'd completely forgotten. Joe calmed down a little and came back and finished up the interview. Then there was a little pause and I leaned in and asked him for a hug, which he gave, somewhat grudgingly. 'Are we buds again?' I said.

It was kind of amazing: my protectiveness of him, my need to feel reassured that he was OK, in spite of everything I'd known even then about his unscrupulousness. It seemed to say something about how he exercised his power, how it rested on a perception of his vulnerability, how he weaponized his own fragility; and it was striking how I had responded to it.

Late November, exact date unknown

I am back in London. I have been remiss keeping the diary, knowing I need to show up for the family and can't expend surplus labour on side projects. It is taking ages for my body clock to return to something like normal and as hard as I try I tend to drift and mope. Maybe I am out of the habit of adjusting to jet lag or maybe it was always this bad. I am all right going to bed. I sleep seven or eight hours, but I feel like a zombie in the morning, like someone walking underwater.

I'd flown back from Dallas, landing at Heathrow at 6.02 a.m., the first plane to touch down that morning. It was hideous. My body was desperate to sleep, thinking it was midnight, as I faced a full day on London time.

Oddly, new rules were just announced that very morning to say self-isolating times will be cut if you get a negative test after five days. 'Test and release.'

The family is intact, and Nancy has been on top of everything. She seemed pleased to see me, which I wasn't sure I could count on. She went off to work and I tried to stay on my feet, doing Zoom calls on development and stories we were working on. I was happy to be back but felt poleaxed and needed to focus quite hard on LOOKING PLEASED to be back and also conscious of the need to hit the ground running with respect to cooking and childcare.

London is still in lockdown – the lockdown reboot or low-fat lockdown, as opposed to the original formula lockdown of March and April. Pubs and many shops are closed but people go to work, they crowd the supermarkets and the parks and the playgrounds. It's hard to tell what the mood is like in the country but in this house, at least, the strain is showing. Around eleven tonight I asked

Jack for his phone. He told me shut up or flip off. I asked again, then broke my rule and just shouted and grabbed it.

Nancy, annoyed, said, 'EVERYONE WAS HAPPIER WHEN YOU WERE AWAY!'

December 2020

RUN AWAY

Thursday 3 December

There is a vaccine. The UK is the first country to approve it. This is the moment we've been waiting for, runs the coverage. This is the soft glow of the coming dawn. Roll-out is being planned. Care workers, NHS staff first. Some are saying the decision has been rushed, including Anthony Fauci, head of US vaccination and health.

Lockdown is technically over but the atmosphere feels very far from triumphalist. Certain football matches can now have partial crowds, likewise small audiences in theatres. Two or three thousand fans at arenas. At a couple of games – Millwall I think and one up north – attendees blessed with the first reappearance at live sports events in nearly nine months used the occasion to boo the players who knelt in recognition of Black Lives Matter.

Saturday 5 December

The day started with the usual routine of football drop-offs for the big boys. Ray is back doing Stagecoach for the first time since Lockdown Two. Nancy picked him up, and on the way back they bought a Christmas tree, which we decorated.

In the evening, we watched *Strictly* musicals night. Comedian Bill Bailey was dancing to *Phantom of the Opera*, army veteran presenter man did some kind of Charleston, vowel-less singer HRVY danced a very accomplished American smooth for twenty-nine points (nine from Craig).

I took Ray up. He was disconsolate that he couldn't be part of the family TV viewing. 'I want to watch with everyone.'

Strictly was followed by a new BBC One quiz format called *The Wheel* presented by Michael McIntyre. A collection of non-optimal celebrity guests spinning around on a carousel, as civilian contestants popped up at random in the middle, then attempted to answer questions, with the advice of whichever celebrity adviser the wheel decided to appoint them. Each celeb has a field of expertise, but their input is sometimes wildly off base, which is the most satisfying part of the format – when the pop music guru is asked, 'How many members of Bananarama were there?' and he confidently says seven. It has the look of a show that had been taped over four or five hours, then cut down to forty-five minutes. Celebs keeping the energy up with lots of hand-waving as they spin round on their eponymous wheel, but with Weltschmerz plainly written on their faces.

It was late when we all went up. I lay in bed and, through Aperol- and Prosecco-glazed eyes, read *Girlvert*, a memoir written by the porn performer Ashley Blue. From other areas of the house, there was a mounting atmosphere of unrest, to do with children's lights going off, or not going off, being unable to sleep, groaning and general malaise, until after several trips back and forth someone – possibly me; OK, yes it was me – royally lost his shit and shouted at the top of his lungs to 'STOP IT! JUST STOP IT! JUST STOP!' It was proper next-level rage, which left me afterwards lying in bed with my heart beating hard, surprised at how upset and out of breath I was. But all quiet after that.

Sunday 6 December

Aargh. Ill and listless. I have lost my voice due to last night's shenanigans. At least it's the weekend. I just hope it comes back tomorrow.

Monday 7 December

Still no voice. And I don't mean a husky voice, I mean none. Nothing. Niente. Rien. Zilch. With the result that today was an embarrassing sequence of Zoom calls during which I had to hold up a sign that said, 'I've Lost My Voice.' I tried plugging in my podcast microphone and whispering into it. It was like one of those Internet videos where a sexy young woman flicks the teeth on a comb or scrunches up crepe paper very close to a microphone. It's called ASMR – Autonomous Sensory Meridian Response. The other metaphor that sprang to mind was the cult leader, barely audible in his messages, appearing before a room full of acolytes who fall silent as he murmurs, 'I think access is going to be key' or 'Jamali Maddix did something on cam girls.' (I actually held up a sign that said this.)

Troubling visions of myself as the Julie Andrews of lockdown podcasting, my career cruelly ended by a mysterious deterioration of the vocal chords rendering me incapable of speech. 'The precise cause of Mr Theroux's condition remains obscure . . .' the reports would say – there was no way I could reveal it was because I'd shouted at the children for not going to bed. Not to mention that I don't have any kind of insurance for workplace injury, so the pay cut would be precipitous, but my own fault I suppose.

We are trying to arrange Christmas. Hoping to have family over, possibly eating in the garden, buffet-style and Covid-safe. Nancy very keen it should happen and to play host to the wider family. But it's still unclear exactly what the rules are and how it will work.

Fucking pangolin. Fucking bloke who ate a pangolin.

Tuesday 8 December

Reports on the radio of the first people getting the vaccine.

Nancy said, 'It would be funny if they came out and they were like, "I feel great!" And there was a second head starting to grow out of their necks.'

'Right, side effects,' I said.

On social media, a ninety-one-year-old man's kerbside interview following his jab was doing the rounds. 'I couldn't find anywhere to park my car . . . I'd had a rather nasty lunch . . . There's no point in dying now, when I've lived this long. I don't plan to anyway.'

In the evening I assembled a collection of leftover dishes – a Mississippi pot roast, a Thai green curry made from chicken rescued from a mustard and vinegar dish from Nigel Slater, Nancy's chickpea Ottolenghi, mashed potato, old salad. It was not 'one of my classics', and there was restiveness coming from below decks.

'I need GRAPES!' Jack said. 'Why can't we go to the Co-op and GET GRAPES!'

'Woah, Jack, way to influence people through charm and positivity. Try a different approach.'

'Please can we go to the supermarket and *get gra-apes*,' he sang.

'That's more like it.'

'Maybe you could offer something in return,' Nancy said to Jack. 'Like offer to clear the table?'

'Good idea,' I said. 'One hand washes the other.'

Jack's face, if I'd seen it, would have said 'cringe'.

Hunched over and mechanical, like a zombie operated by remote control, he lurched round the table, picked up a single pepper pot, cleared it, then returned for a single bowl.

'I don't think much of the waiter, do you?' I said.

'He seems like he might be on drugs.'

Later that night, after I'd put Ray down and read two Christmas stories and we'd watched episode four of the *Star Wars* space western, *The Mandalorian*, I was tidying in the kitchen. It was eleven or so. 'Time to go up, Jack,' I said. *Groan.* 'Can I have the phone and I can charge it?'

He handed it over without fuss. Progress. When I followed him upstairs I found him sprawled on his bed.

'Can you put toothpaste on my toothbrush, Dad?' he said.

'Seriously?'

'Please,' he said. 'I gave you my phone.'

As I left to do it, he said, 'One hand washes the other.'

Wednesday 9 December

Voice slightly coming back, dark brown version.

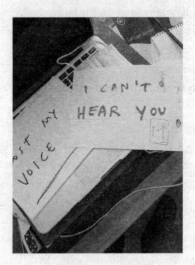

Zoom accessories.

Friday 11 December

At Ray's drop-off, a girl in his class gave him a hug. Her mother is Italian.

'She said that Ray told her he can speak Spanish, but he can't remember any words. She was a bit confused.'

An email has come in from the campaigner Peter Tatchell, forwarding a message he received from Jeremy Bamber's team in which they lay out, point by point, a set of complaints they have about our production. We've been on the outs with the Bamber team for some weeks, for reasons that are frustrating because they seem rooted in misunderstandings brought on by the distance enforced on us by the pandemic. For more than a year, we've been in touch and they've been on board with the idea of working with us on the series, but now that's all changed. Bamber himself, who was due to be interviewed for the series – one conversation had already taken place – is now off the menu. I'd hoped we might salvage the relationship. But the message to Peter suggests otherwise. From somewhere, they have heard that we are 'anti-Bamber'. In fact, we have been attempting to be studiously even-handed, keeping an open mind as to whether there might have been a miscarriage of justice. It is enormously stressful. We keep on – we have no other choice. I called Peter to explain the background. He is still up for an interview. He says he will try to help mend relations with the Bamber team.

In some good news, my voice is now something approaching normal.

A text from our TV Insider Friend to say London is going into tier three on Wednesday. Nancy said she'd already heard rumours.

Saturday 12 December

Gloomy and rainy.

In the evening Nancy and I took the tube down to Brixton. The train was half full. Almost everyone wearing masks.

'Can you imagine if you had a vision of this, this time last year? What you would think?' Nancy said.

With a little distance it seemed very weird.

Tuesday 15 December

London and the south-east are in tier three from midnight tonight. You can go into a shop if it has an entry point on the ground floor. Tattoo parlours open. Pubs not open. Hairdressers I'm not sure. On the radio, complaints that lockdown has gone too far and also that it hasn't gone far enough. People indignant at others who are indignant back at them, others indignant at lack of indignation. Me mainly indignant at indignation overload.

Jack said this morning that he didn't need to go into school today.

'What?' Nancy said.

Arthur had been off school since yesterday.

'Everyone at school said, there was no school.'

'I would have got a message. Louis, what are you doing?'

I was checking my Fantasy Football score on my phone.

'I'm checking the school website,' I said. The school website had announcements about prizes and inspection reports and pictures of children playing ball games and holding up paintings but nothing I could see relevant to the question of whether they were admitting children.

'Oh, there is a message,' Nancy said. 'For fuck's sake.'

Jack had already left, gone upstairs, without eating any breakfast.

In the evening, Nancy and I went out for a farewell-to-freedom drink and meal at a restaurant in Queen's Park with our TV Insider Friend, the same one who had told me we would be entering tier three days before it happened, and who always has intel on what's coming next. His view is that we'll be in this for many more months.

'Edinburgh Festival will be remote next year,' he said. 'Who wants to be with 3,000 people elbow-to-elbow in an auditorium?'

'What about the vaccine?'

'Forget it,' Nancy said. 'There's no way they'll have enough people vaccinated.'

'I think they might.'

'What, this government? Forget it.'

Wednesday 16 December

The virus is surging in America and the UK and it now looks as though the government was rash to suppose that we could get together at Christmas in various bubble configurations. They haven't changed the rules again – though many want them to. But they are discouraging excessive mingling.

I was driving down to the Co-op on an emergency grapes and milk run, listening to the radio. A government man said, *'It's like a speed limit. If the road is icy, you know to keep well below it.'*

Reasonable analogy, whoever you are, I thought.

Jack was at home again today. Was he working? Who knows? He has decided he wants to take up skateboarding. At lunchtime he and Arthur were talking cordially over their pasta pesto about TikTok or some video game update or Red Dead online, then got up to clear their plates and started arguing over who had had too many chocolates from the other's Advent calendar. It escalated quickly to major batten-down-the-hatches ranting and raving. I drifted ineffectually from room to room.

In the afternoon, I did a remote corporate Q & A for a tech company whose line of work I didn't really understand. I'd been sent a kitbag of lights and a phone and tripods. Assembling the kit was like an IQ test or an espionage assignment. Laminated instruction cards. 'In a plastic pouch you will find a disinfected iPhone charged and pre-loaded with an app. You need to update the app. There are two AirPods. Assemble the three tripods and make sure your background is free of clutter.'

I was losing the will to live and starting to panic at the same time. I'd allowed myself forty-five minutes prep time but it didn't seem enough. I could practically hear the bomb defusal danger music speeding up in my head. Then I was joined remotely by a husband-and-wife team eight time zones away in Topanga Canyon who directed me at long distance.

'Left light . . . down a bit . . . A bit more orange? And more? Split the difference.'

'We're seeing too much door.'

'I'm more worried about the colour temperature.'

'What if we go left, I'm just wondering about the filing cabinet.'

I sensed they had been spending a lot of time together and might be on the verge of an argument.

Once the Q & A began, possibly tripping on adrenaline, I went into Lockdown Guru mode, pontificating about the State of the World, offering advice, and weirdly starting to believe my own ravings about Covid and learning from adversity and 'getting Theroux' it, coming off like Tony Robbins auditioning for a Nobel Peace Prize. I was being interviewed by a woman called Clare who was also in her own home, in Ireland, and halfway through my Manifesto for a New Humanity I could hear the grinding bass of drill music coming from downstairs. Jack was on the smart speaker. 'Humans crave connection,' I said. *Wet you up with my shank.* 'Those moments we recall with most pleasure are challenges we overcame.' *Spill that claret. Make that ting go blat-blat-blat!* Luckily it was inaudible to the production team and to Clare.

Thursday 17 December

An announcement on the radio. There will be staggered opening next year for secondary schools for years that aren't taking exams in the summer. Which would be our two big guys. Also, a get-together on the twenty-third with Mum and Michael is postponed because Michael's vaccine won't have taken effect yet.

What phase of the pandemic are we at? More places going into tier three. Families being 'discouraged' from meeting in large groups. Christmas isn't cancelled but Prancer has had his antlers clipped and Santa's baubles are in the nutcracker.

Ray's nativity play has been posted online. *The Jolly Postman*. He played the part of a wolf, within an ensemble of wolves with seven or eight other children. The other groups were gingerbread men and bears. We were all sent links. I tried to watch it in the kitchen with Nancy, while making supper at the same time.

'Louis, are you watching?'

'You start, I'll be right there.'

When I joined I was pleased to see Ray was giving it 100 per cent, the effect only slightly diminished by buffering issues. '*Ho ho ho! I'm a jolly little wolf . . .*' Buffering again. '*Aooh! I'm a wolfie-wolfie-wolf,*' More buffering. The good part was, with the advantage of editing and multiple takes, there was no mumbling or interminable waiting as children shuffled on and off stage.

'I think the nativity play is actually slightly better in the Covid version,' I said. 'It's tighter and you don't have to watch the other children.'

When I went to take Ray upstairs, he was watching the latest in a series on YouTube called 'How To Survive . . .' (a zombie attack; a house fire; running out of oxygen in space). He had a little notebook with a few things scrawled in it in pencil. Upstairs he realized he'd forgotten his notebook and asked me to get it. On the way back up, I looked inside. There were only two words. 'Run away.'

I wrote my diary in my room, which still had its weird klieg lights left over from the corporate – I'd kept them up because I felt they gave me the edge in Zoom calls. I liked being well lit and it gave me an enjoyable sense of performance, like I was a superstar at life. Nancy called from downstairs and I came down – Art had been watching *Peaky Blinders* but he wasn't in a good mood. Jack came over eating a brownie.

'What are you eating?' Art asked.

Jack didn't answer.

'What are you eating?'

'A brownie I made. It's the last one.'

Jack was just wearing some tight boxers.

'Why are you just wearing boxers?'

'It's not a big deal, is it, Art?' I said. 'Someone wandering around in boxers?'

Art stood up and went upstairs.

'I can hear him crying,' Nancy said. Then she said, 'I don't know how to get through any more lockdown stuff. I just don't.'

Monday 21 December

And just like that the government has U-turned and London and the south-east have gone into tier four. To be honest, I didn't know the tiers went that high. There will be no mixing at Christmas, no guests, no indoor mingling and cracker pulling: our entire Christmas scenario, lovingly envisioned and planned towards by Nancy, has been banjaxed. This all because of a 'new variant' of the virus, which does not make people crave human flesh, and is not more deadly, but *is* apparently more contagious and affects children. So they tell us. You can only leave the house for specific purposes or if you have a 'reasonable excuse'. Shopping for essentials and work that cannot be done at home. Outdoors you can meet one person from another household. Indoors, only someone from an existing support bubble.

Today I took the kids for a dental appointment in Harlesden. In the evening, in a crisis Zoom conference, Nancy's family picked through the debris of the plan for the Christmas get-together, debating whether there might be a workaround that involved dropping off gifts outside at people's front doors or maybe socializing at distance in a green space or on pavements. Nancy, who has already ordered a turkey big enough to feed twenty-five and had her heart set on having people over, grew upset as it became clear no one would be visiting and left the Zoom, walked off screen, without ending the call, and so it went on in the background. I'd been upstairs putting Ray down and when I came into the kitchen she was crying in the corner and I could hear the conference still going on, the tinny sound of their voices debating coming from the computer at the end of the table, commiserating over Nancy's disappointment, and wondering what was safe and what the right thing to do was. I went over and hugged her and told her it would be OK.

'We'll still have a nice Christmas, Nancy,' I said. 'Ernesto's still coming and maybe in a funny way it will end up being more memorable and special.'

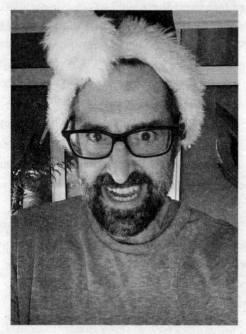

Government elf warning.

Wednesday 23 December

Zoomed with my friends Joe and Adam. It's a tradition dating back to our early twenties that we have an evening drink together on Christmas Eve – we used to do it back when we all lived with our respective parents in South London. I'd cycle round to Adam's house and Joe would join and we'd raise a glass with Adam's dad, Nigel, whose courtly old-world sensibilities made us giggle but whose presence also had a civilizing effect on our conversation. We'd talk about his days as the Travel Editor of the *Daily Telegraph* and about the alcoholic newsreader of the seventies, Reggie Bosanquet, whom Nigel had known. It's been years since we observed the old tradition but I thought it might be nice to resurrect it in lockdown, remotely, on the eve of Christmas Eve.

I was delayed a few minutes, noticing as I came upstairs that our bed was covered in presents, which I quickly removed and stacked neatly on the floor. Then I went up to the top floor and fired up the computer. Joe came on first, then Adam joined and we made chit-chat about life and Covid and spun off into a conversational side alley about a comedy-writer friend who has found a second calling as a feminist scourge of what he considers trans overreach, fighting an insurgent war on Twitter, until he was kicked off it, to the point where he has lost friends and work. Joe's eyes were glazing over. He has a young child and was tired. Soon after he said goodnight, and then I chatted with Adam until I heard sounds of outrage from downstairs. 'Louis! Those presents were organized! What were you *thinking*?' I hurriedly said goodnight.

Thursday 24 December

A marathon of gift wrapping, which I was doing in the bedroom while listening to a podcast about catching Internet paedophiles, called *Hunting Warhead*. Nancy kept coming in and switching it back to Christmas music, and then I'd switch it back to the paedophile podcast. I guess that was the sort of mood I was in. I did a Joe Wicks around 5 p.m. to clear my head. The last couple of days there's been a mounting background feeling of apocalypticism. Intimations of schools not going back in January, further tightening of the rules, a new strain that's popped up here, the South Africa variant, in addition to the other new strain, the Kent variant.

In the late afternoon Uncle Ernesto arrived, self-advertised Covid renegade. He is a single man and we are his support bubble, so technically it is allowed. Nancy and I opened a bottle of Prosecco. Having done my Joe Wicks I was feeling virtuous. I poured myself some bourbon. Ernesto is a fan of a certain kind of high-octane one-man-against-the-world action film. It's part of family lore that his favourite movie is *First Blood* and on his Facebook page he used to feature a favourite quote from the protagonist John Rambo, which was, 'To kill. Period.' For a while he was studying to be a doctor and I used to joke that he should have the quote on the business card of his medical practice. He asked the boys if they'd ever seen *Die Hard*, which they hadn't, so we put it on and watched, as I scuttled back and forth to the kitchen topping up my bourbon and lemon juice and soda.

'I think you've had enough to drink,' Nancy said.

'Tea anyone?' I asked.

I went out and poured myself another one, but kept the glass in the sink so she wouldn't see it if she came in. I did this twice, aware as it was happening that it was not a good sign on any level – for what it said about my drinking or about my relationship. 'You're only as sick as your secrets,' as they say in AA. Around midnight I had a last bourbon, washing down a Nurofen with it, then went up and read *Lambs to the Slaughter*, a true-crime account of a notorious paedophile ring that operated in Hackney in the eighties, trying to figure out if there might be a way to tell the story on TV, though most of the culprits are dead, and also aware that through the bourbon haze I might not be thinking clearly. At one in the morning I went to sleep.

Friday 25 December

Up at 7.30, zombified, barely able to raise a smile as I watched the children opening their stockings and cooing over their toys. All day I found weird things irritating that I shouldn't have. Questions about the turkey and meandering Zoom calls with family talking across one another and Christmas songs and 'Stay Another Day' by East 17. 'He seems very sinister,' I heard myself say, apropos of one of the members of that completely innocuous boy group. I was bent on pouring poison on a blameless world. 'I hate that song. It brims with an aggressive inanity. It exudes darkness. *Stay another day!*' In the afternoon, we had a socially distanced accidental-on-purpose 'bump-into' with one of Nancy's brothers and their family in Queen's Park. We exchanged a couple of gifts and stood around in the cold wet park for an hour or so. Nancy's brother said he was feeling ill but didn't have a cough so it wasn't Covid. I was his Secret Santa and handed over his gifts, a graphic novel I thought he would enjoy and some award-winning luxury marmalade.

I seem to hate everything. I think I must be in a bad mood. Happy Christmas.

Sunday 27 December

Today, on WhatsApp, Nancy's brother, who we'd met in the park, announced he has tested positive for Covid. Long discussion this evening about what we do now, Arthur chipping in with readings of the rules. We were trying to recall if he'd hugged Nancy at some point. I'd given him his gift but I hadn't got close and definitely hadn't hugged him.

'Surely the whole of his family will get it?' I said.

'Well, some people have immunity. It depends on your T-cells,' Nancy said.

Feels weird having it close to home. Earlier in the day, Ernesto had said, 'What was the mortality rate of the bubonic plague?'

'Er, don't know.'

'Eighty per cent.'

'Ooh. What about Covid?'

'0.02 per cent.' Whether this is the true statistic, no one seems to know. I googled it later. Others say 0.2.

In the evening we watched *Die Hard* 2 with Ernesto and I finished reading my book about the 1980s paedophile ring. Feeling vaguely unsettled or maybe ill.

Wednesday 30 December

Nancy got tested. She is negative for corona. I made a leftover turkey pie for freezing. In the afternoon I watched *ParaNorman* with Ray and tried to nap.

I don't want to leave the house or make arrangements.

The *New York Post* has editorialized against Trump's refusal to concede. 'STOP THE INSANITY – You lost the election – here's how to save your legacy.' Covid is off the charts in the UK. Hospitals overrun. They announced that primary schools are not going back in the new year. Nancy depressed and upset. Me weirdly blank and resigned.

Thursday 31 December

In the morning, I did a little work on the Joe Exotic film, then came downstairs and in the fridge spied the little plastic pouch that had come with the Christmas turkey, containing the giblets, languishing unloved, a little grotesque, possibly on the turn. I'd noticed them before, and had meant to put them to use – was it too late? I googled and found a recipe for turkey liver mousse and another for braised turkey neck, and a third for fried turkey heart. Jack and I followed the recipes – finding most of the supporting cast of ingredients, the cream and white wine, in the fridge. We ate the heart first and then for lunch the neck, shredded in brioche buns, and the mousse with cornichons. 'Pretty good, right, Jack?' I said. 'Delicious,' he replied, and in what I suppose was the ultimate tribute to the meal refused to let Arthur have any.

Didn't leave the house in daylight.

In the evening we looked over the fence at the neighbours' fireworks and raised a remote toast. At 11 p.m. Nancy and I put the TV on. BBC Two was showing an episode of *Before They Were Famous* presented by Angus Deayton. Seeing Angus Deayton was the first surprise. I couldn't recall seeing him present anything in years. One of the celebrities was a singer in Steps. There was also footage of Patsy Palmer in a zit-cream commercial and Ross Kemp *with hair* doing an instructional video about customer service in a DIY store. Then it dawned on me the programme was a rerun, and had originally aired fifteen, maybe twenty years ago. It was vaguely paradoxical: an old programme featuring celebrities wearing out-of-date clothes and haircuts making jokes about the clothes and haircuts of other celebrities in clips that were even older.

BBC One was showing a new *Graham Norton* but they were all sitting far apart, or guests were calling in via Zoom, and it was all too redolent of Covid so we switched over to Channel 5 which had on a three-hour-long countdown show called *Fifty Favourite Singles from the Eighties*. The Bangles' 'Eternal Flame'. 'Karma Chameleon'. I had opened a third or fourth bottle of Prosecco and I was enjoying it all, if anything, a little too much, the vision of an era of bright colours and primitive special effects and great music. The kids were double screening, engrossed in their phones but seemingly happy just to be sharing a room with us. At number one was 'Last Christmas' by Wham. By now it was one in the morning. Nancy said it was time to turn in. I lurched upstairs and lay in bed with the bedside lamp on, finding in my hand a copy of my memoir *Gotta Get Theroux This*. I must have been pissed because I began reading it and enjoying it.

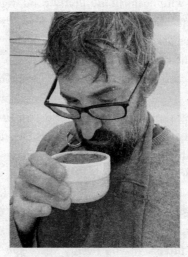

We are not amoussed.

January 2021

DINOSAUR MOMENT

Friday 1 January

In the afternoon, we went for a long walk with friends who live in Hampstead. Halfway through, finding the walk too long for his tastes, Ray revolted, took his coat off and stamped on it, then sat on the muddy ground, groaning and complaining. We were lagging behind the group, which paused then moved on, not wishing to intrude on an embarrassing display. I tried to negotiate, then hoisted him up and carried him on my shoulders, trudging through the twilight like an old cottager lugging winter fuel. I'm a fifty-year-old man. When my dad was this age, his youngest son was twenty. I know because it was me.

Yesterday was the highest daily death toll in the US to date: 3,462.

This evening, Nancy discovered we might qualify as key workers because we make programmes for the BBC, i.e. a public service broadcaster. Meaning Ray might be able to go back to school after all. Please God.

Thursday 7 January

Lockdown Three definitely turning out to be my least favourite of the trilogy. Unoriginal plot, crap special effects. You'd think the writers would want to mix it up a bit after the disappointment of Lockdown Two. But if anything they've gone *more* grim and sucked out any of the remaining joie de vivre. A bit like Christopher Nolan with the second *Dark Knight* film.

The latest measures were announced yesterday. Kids not going back until after half term. More home schooling, though Ray will go in three days a week. No children's football. Various productions we have been working on now thrown into doubt.

Morale is low, in this heart anyway. I feel like going to bed at 8.30. They say the hospitals are being overrun. Too many elderly and frontline health workers incapacitated. A relentless slow-moving tsunami of the critically ill. Positive tests are off the charts. Daily death in the UK: 874 yesterday. Close to what it was at the height of the pandemic. It's said they can keep people alive now, but it creates a log jam in hospitals, which is a lovely image: a log jam of insensate, supine Covid-sufferers wedged together in a corridor.

In the morning I had a monster argument with Nancy for obscure reasons. She was getting stressed because the cleaners were coming and went into nag-mode. Yes, I just wrote that. I'd been up early with Ray and he was acting up, whining and crying. I tried to conciliate him by sitting with him and playing cards and Deblok, a puzzle game involving patterned cubes, instead of attending to the mess in the kitchen. Nancy came down and saw this and gave no quarter.

'So you haven't emptied the dishwasher?'

'No,' I said, and then figuring it was better to go on the offensive, I said, 'Why do you act as though I do nothing around the house?'

It escalated quickly, which was not ideal, especially since the kids were upstairs and could hear.

I spent the day on Zoom calls, then picked up Ray from school. News was coming in that both Senate seats in Georgia had gone to the Democrat candidates, giving Biden control of the Senate. I had a bourbon and made supper while listening to a rough cut of the Twigs chat from several months ago. It sounded pretty good. I had a couple more bourbons to celebrate.

Trumpers were converging on Washington DC, egged on by the Orange Man. The bourbon was kicking in and I was feeling relaxed. Nancy put Ray to bed, and I plonked myself down in the TV room on my favourite chair to watch the latest Attenborough on catch-up. The TV was showing a frog that was literally frozen, with ice over its eyeballs, which then came back to life. It seemed like one of the most extraordinary things I'd ever seen on television and several times I heard myself say 'Wow, that is *unbelievable*', and I was thinking if you saw this on drugs you would think you were hallucinating.

'Are you drunk?' Nancy asked.

'No, but you've got to admit that was amazing. The frog was literally frozen.'

All this time my phone was pinging with incoming WhatsApp messages from the group that was looking into our long-gestating story on dissident right-wingers. In Washington DC, Trumpers had apparently invaded the Capitol building and several of our prospective contributors were involved. One, called Baked Alaska, had posted a selfie of himself in a congressional office, and in the background was a guy who looked like Nick Fuentes, the far-right leader we were meant to film in March last year.* Twitter was going loco

* The man in the background was later revealed to be someone else, not Fuentes.

but I wasn't clear-headed enough to figure out exactly what was happening. There was a sense of historic outrage, an unprecedented cataclysm, which is to say, it was possibly just another day in the Twitterverse. I scrolled my phone: the sight of what looked like unwashed hordes storming the cradle of American democracy was pretty weird, but then again was it as weird as a frog that can freeze and then come back to life?

Recalling that there was a pile of washing-up in the sink, I headed to the kitchen to load the dishwasher, though maybe a more persuasive reason to go in there was that I would be unsupervised and could have another drink. I squeezed more lemons and poured out more bourbon with soda water. I'd made myself a semi-rule to only drink between six and ten and it was ten thirty now. But when I ran a quick audit of my systems the verdict came back: *not that pissed*. No harm in another one. By now I'd also heard from Nancy that Oliver Stone had sent a nice Instagram message about how much he'd enjoyed our interview, so that was another cause for celebration.

I put some music on, a mix I'd made in 2017, and found myself dancing around the room, and wondering what it might be like to go on *Strictly Come Dancing*. Could I win? Bill Bailey had won and he was an older man. What would Craig Revel Horwood say? I'd have to get even more fit, that was half the battle. But then, Bill Bailey didn't look that fit. I did robot moves to some US electronica. It would be nice to have another drink but I also allowed that it was a Wednesday. Like a mountaineer in the death zone, with a turnback time that he no longer wants to stick to, my clouded head told me I was supposed to stop, reverse course, but I really wanted to keep climbing and that seemed much more important.

After that it's a little bit of a blur. I may have had another drink. The dishwasher had broken down mid-cycle so I pulled it out of the wall to see if that helped. Was music played? Another drink? The camera spins around and points at the ceiling and defocuses as it zooms in on a bulb . . .

I awoke surprised to find myself in the spare bed in Jack's room and a blank spot where the end of the night should have been. I didn't feel hungover. I felt a little weird, though. Maybe still a little drunk? I tried to remember the end of the evening but there wasn't much there other than a dim memory of lying next to Nancy and trying to read an article on my phone in the dark and that it kept making loud noises and maybe she'd asked me to leave.

I went downstairs. Nancy was already up. 'You feeling OK?' she said with a knowing tone.

'Not too bad.' I didn't actually feel that bad.

For a second I was taken aback to find the dishwasher standing in the middle of the kitchen, looking faintly surreal, like the detritus from a hurricane. On the radio the news was all about the Capitol invasion, which according to some commentators had been a kind of putsch staged by Trump in a fit of pique about losing the election. While I'd been marvelling at a frog that could freeze and then come back to life, Trump had allegedly been attempting a half-cocked coup d'état. That was the narrative anyway, though seizing power by unleashing an unruly mob of the lumpenproletariat on the US Capitol seems an ill-thought-out plan at best. Don't you need high-level military onside or a revolutionary vanguard, as prescribed by nineteenth-century professional revolutionary Louis Blanqui? Commentators were lining up to denounce Trump's crowd-based eructation as a shameful moment of anti-democratic sedition. Foreign leaders were piling in. A protester, an army vet called Ashli Babbitt, had been shot and killed trying to force her way into the Capitol. At least three other people were dead but it wasn't clear how. Reported as 'medical emergencies' – a stroke, a heart attack – which I guess is what happens when the over-fifties decide to riot. Members of Congress had been evacuated from the house floor in see-through plastic disposable gas masks. Trump had been paying lip service to 'peacefulness' and had eventually encouraged protesters to 'go home' while also saying 'We love you'.

On Twitter, images from the insurrection were trending and they were like a manifestation of Trump's inner being. Red-eyed cabin folk in plaid and unfashionable jeans. One photo that went viral showed a self-advertised shaman, shirtless and tribal-tattooed and wearing a bison-headdress complete with horns – he looked the spit of late-nineties-era Jamiroquai frontman Jay Kay – while others showed guys, mostly white, bearded, whooping in the rotunda, some in full paramilitary garb.

The hangover kicked in late morning. It wasn't crippling, just debilitating and depressing, coming on like a slow poison. I joined Twigs for a follow-up Zoom interview – she had wanted to speak again, after coming out as a survivor of alleged physical abuse and coercive control at the hands of her ex, the actor Shia LaBoeuf, which he denies. I felt like an invalid coming round from a coma, though still focused enough to have the conversation, which ended up having a tonic effect owing to her poise and thoughtfulness. Afterwards, I managed a Joe Wicks, which helped further, then in the evening, no drink, herbal tea only. We watched Attenborough again. This time: baby turtles emerging from their underground eggs, just hatched, drowning because the rains had come too early, because of climate change.

Jack: 'They don't *know* that's because of climate change.'

Attenborough, seconds later: 'It's happening because of changes in the climate . . .'

Friday 8 January

The UK announced its worst figures for coronavirus deaths, 1,325, exactly fourteen days since Christmas and the one-day relaxation of rules.

Art has elected to go to school on-site, which he can do thanks to our key worker status, which has come through, and which, yes, I feel a little weird about. But evidently there's room. He did his second on-site school day, which he said he enjoyed. Jack doesn't want to go in. So he'll still be remote learning. Or possibly not remote learning.

This time last year I was touring Australia playing to crowds seated elbow to elbow, aerosolizing willy-nilly. Remember those days?

Trump gave a speech denouncing the riots for 'defiling' the people's house. Many high-level Republicans peeling away. Talk of impeachment or invoking the twenty-fifth amendment for mental incapacity. Some resignations from members of his cabinet. Nancy Pelosi has vowed to impeach. But polls show half of Republicans are still on board with him. I check Twitter to see what the right-wingers are saying. Eric and Don Jr. both denounced the violence. Trump-supporting actor James Woods – literally nothing on it. Ted Cruz on the radio saying he disagrees with 'Trump's rhetoric.' Scott Adams, the Dilbert guy, seems mainly upset that Trump apologized. Some are suggesting that because a BLM guy was spotted at the protests that they were behind it. The right and the libertarian left make pro forma condemnations of the violence, then pivot to suggest that because Trump has been banned from Twitter the real problem is the prospect of an Orwellian tech industry that purges heretics and freethinkers from their platforms and stifles dissent.

At supper, we ordered a Thai. A meal, not a human. We talked about Ashli Babbitt, the air force vet who was killed in the Capitol. Her social media footprint has revealed her to have been a sometime Obama voter turned QAnon believer. Art said he'd seen footage of her being shot.

'It wasn't that bad,' Jack said. 'You couldn't see anything.'

'Is it on YouTube?' I asked.

'It's everywhere,' Jack said.

Art said, 'On TikTok, some people were saying, "Well you made fun of BLM deaths so we're going to make fun of that woman's death" and they did comedy videos around it.'

'That's horrible.'

'Why did they storm a BTEC White House?' Jack asked. 'Why didn't they just storm the White House?'

'Because Trump is in the White House and they're Trump supporters.'

Sunday 10 January

On a drive to St James's Park we listened to Capital Xtra. This is our default station since it's the only one Jack will tolerate. The main diet is drill, grime, some US hip hop, and a handful of older rap and R&B tracks. Though he likes it, Jack gets irked if we enjoy it *too much*. He also doesn't like it if we express interest in a track or recognize an artist. 'Isn't this Headie One?' 'I like this one. Is it Buggzy?' etc. On the other hand, if you ask to change it, he is liable to say, as he did on this occasion, 'What, so we can listen to *Bob Lennon*?'

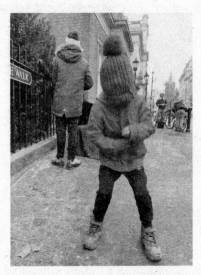

Six-year-old with improvised face covering.

Wednesday 13 January

'Substantial' risk of intensive care beds running out, admits Johnson. That's the headline in *The Times*. The US also suffered its worst day ever. 'But this summer could be "dramatically better",' says CNN.

We all seem to know that the summer will be better. In the UK, the rise in infections is showing signs of slowing and 2.25 million first doses of the vaccine have been administered. They are doing 1.3 million a week. But it feels bleak and everyone now either has had it or knows someone who has had it. Two colleagues at work have it, though neither very seriously. Cold symptoms basically, someone said.

Thursday 14 January

It was Year 8 parents' evening. At twelve minutes past four Jack and I sat in front of my laptop trying to log on. It kept failing to get through to the page. I texted Nancy, who was on a Zoom call. I tried a different browser. I cursed myself for leaving it too late. Several minutes went by. For each subject there was a five-minute window. We were now late for the design and technology teacher. I tried again. I texted Nancy. Now we were late for the science teacher.

Jack, who had his phone, said: 'There's a problem with the system.' The page loaded, finally, but no teacher came on.

'They've given up,' Jack said. 'They're rescheduling for another time.'

'Well, that was a waste of half an hour,' I said.

Earlier in the day, Art came back from school saying he'd been sent home and had to self-isolate for two days. I had been recording links in my office for the Leah Remini episode of the podcast.

'The boy who sits next to me tested positive,' Art said.

'Oh dear. I'm just on a call . . .'

'I tested negative.'

'Oh, OK.'

'But I still have to self-isolate,' he said.

'OK.'

He stopped on the stairs. 'Also, Dad? I'm really sorry. That hat you like? The boy with coronavirus touched it so I put a sign there. Don't touch it.'

At supper, I said, 'So what happens now? Does he have to stay in his room? Is it like in *Ben Hur* with the lepers, and we have to put his meals through a little hatch in the door?'

Nancy said, 'We're not going to put him in isolation in his room. *He tested negative.*'

Either way, Art has to stay at home for a few days.

Supper was a leftover turkey pie I'd made weeks ago and frozen. Jack arrived late, saw the pie and the mash.

'Not eating that,' he said and left.

'Jack, you come back here at once!' Nancy said.

'I'm not eating that.'

'Your dad has made a delicious Jamie Oliver pie and you're being very rude.'

'He had a bowl of cereal probably half an hour ago so he may not be hungry,' I said.

'At least you can sit with your family.'

Jack sat and ate some pie. But no mashed potato.

After supper, Jack asked if we could go to the Co-op. I was feeling frazzled and realized I hadn't left the house all day.

'We can go to the Co-op if we walk.'

'OK,' he said.

Outside it was dark and cold and damp. I set off at a clip.

'Come on,' I said.

'Why are you going so fast?'

'It's good exercise.'

'If you go that fast I'll just go back.'

'Fine, I'll slow down. What's your favourite movie, do you think?' I asked.

'Don't know. I know my favourite TV show. It's called *Attack on Titan*. It's anime.'

'Would you like to go to Japan one day?'

'Yeah,' he said.

'Maybe we could go on holiday. When this is all over.'

We walked on past Brondesbury Park station, over the road, skipping puddles. The streets were clear and in the dark you could see inside other homes, where the curtain weren't closed – people watching TV, standing in their kitchens, leading their lives.

Friday 15 January

Ray wasn't at school, it being a Friday, so I helped him out on his Zoom learning. There's some progress now. There's a little bit of a sense that they may be learning something. Ray said hello to the classmates then muted himself again.

'Shall we play the mute game?' the teacher said. 'Mohammed, Simon says *unmute*.'

In the afternoon I tried to get him to make a collage or a mosaic out of some old bits of china we'd found at low tide on a Thames walk, but there wasn't that much, so I'd dug out an old jam jar with sea glass in it. *This is classic dad stuff*, I'd thought. *I'll win Dad of the Year. We'll make a seascape, the sea glass will be the sea, and the china will be some kind of boat.*

I found an old shoe box in the recycling to make a case for the mosaic.

'Ray, do you want to make a mosaic out of the treasure?'

'NOOO!'

After Ray had gone up, Nancy watched *The Circle* on Channel 4 with the big boys while I wrote my diary. Then, in bed, after the lights went off, I hugged Nancy.

'I'm really struggling,' she said.

Saturday 16 January

We cycled down to the park – me, Jack, Nancy and Ray. Nancy was meeting her Yoga Instructor Friend. I stood resolutely two metres away as I said hello, more as a piece of hygiene theatre than anything else.

Yoga Friend said, 'You can't get it outside. It's been proven.'

'You also can't get it from surfaces,' Nancy said. 'That's bullshit.'

'If I sneezed on a surface and you licked the surface you wouldn't get it?' I said.

Nancy sighed. 'I don't know why he's like this.'

Yoga Friend mentioned she had a friend who'd been at the Capitol insurrection. 'American guy, I knew him at LSE. It's very sad.'

'Intelligent?'

'It's almost like he was too intelligent? He was left-wing but he began questioning everything. He tipped over the edge.'

'What did he do?'

'Massage therapist.'

'That'll do it. Was it QAnon?'

'No, I think he just began distrusting everything. I emailed him a while ago and said I think you need to get off social media. He said, "You're projecting. I think *you* need to get off social media." He was very gentle . . . He didn't go inside the building.'

'We need to get our steps in,' Nancy said. 'We're trying to get to 10,000.'

When they got back, Nancy was excited. 'You'll never guess who we saw,' she said. 'Matt Hancock!'

'No! The Health Secretary? What was he doing?'

'He was covered in mud. Carrying a rugby ball. With his son.'

'Maybe he lives around here.'

'He looked younger than I expected,' Yoga Friend said. 'It was a bit annoying.'

'He's probably only thirty-five. Well, forty-five.'

'I wanted to say something to him,' Nancy said.

'What would you say? "Covid lies!" "Stop the Steal!"'

'Well, he was with his son. But I would have said, "Tory cunt."'

When we got home, there was a headline in the Mail Online: 'Matt Hancock filmed out in London park after Boris Johnson's national plea to "stay home this weekend" – as crowds flock to beauty spots, supermarket shoppers refuse to wear masks and anti-lockdown protesters are arrested.'

In the evening, we watched a horror film called *Don't Breathe*. Three young burglars break into a house belonging to a blind Gulf War vet who turns out to be a deranged sadist who imprisons and terrorizes them. As an older man, with three young people imprisoned in my house, I found myself identifying more with the psychopath than with the burglars.

'I actually want him to shoot those Hollywood yuppie burglars,' I said.

Nancy wasn't having it. 'You're rooting for the psychopath who has a woman imprisoned in his basement?'

'He has PTSD from Iraq and she ran over his daughter. Which doesn't excuse it, but the point is, they didn't know he had a woman in his basement when they broke in. So I am *not* rooting for those kids.'

'OK, you're drunk,' Nancy said. 'And you are spoiling the film now. So please shut up.'

Monday 18 January

From one of Nancy's brothers, a message: **Hatt Mancock self-isolating. I hope you guys didn't get close to him at the weekend.**

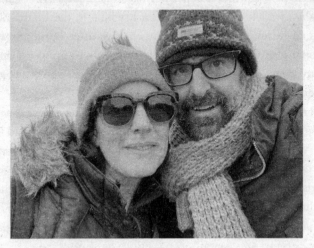

My beautiful wife with a creepy old man.

Wednesday 20 January

Trump's last day as president. In accordance with tradition, in one of his last acts, he embarked upon an orgy of pardoning, extending clemency to a reported 140 people, including the rappers Lil Wayne and Kodak Black and the dark-arts strategist Steve Bannon. For Tiger King Joe Exotic, however – whose team announced they were 100 per cent confident and went so far as to park a stretch limo outside the prison to whisk him away when the pardon came – there is bupkis. It's strange to reflect on the nine months we've had of *Tiger King* mania. Joe's celebrity continues at a high baseline even now, so long after the Netflix series first aired. I have him on Google alerts and every day brings a new story (he's ill, he's in isolation, he's made an 'emotional appeal' to his husband Dylan) and I have to remind myself that he is a real person, someone I knew and was a little bit fond of, not a fictional character, and I wonder whether he considers the global fame he now enjoys as being worth the price of incarceration.

Trump has been seemingly AWOL since January 6 and his permanent muzzling on Twitter. Without his social media bullhorn, he is oddly without impact – there is only, in the conspicuous silence, a memory of the noise, like a leaf blower being turned off.

In the wake of the Twitter ban, Trump was deplatformed from a swathe of social media companies, including the e-commerce company Shopify and an obscure indie film website where fans can post their own reviews. Had he ever used it? Trump-related memes feature a fifteen-year-old girl who was banned from her devices last year, and who figured out how to tweet from her Wii U, then, having been banned from *that*, sent a tweet seemingly from her LG smart fridge, saying: 'I do not know if this is going to tweet I am talking to my fridge what the heck my Mom confiscated all of my electronics again.' I looked it up and there is some debate about whether the girl really did tweet from her fridge. It may be fake news.

There are also stories in the papers alleging Trump has been abandoned by his populist peers in Europe – Duda in Poland, Orbán in Hungary, Matteo Salvini and Marine Le Pen all either decrying the violence at the Capitol or silent.

Much of the coverage since the event at the Capitol carries a triumphalist undertone. As if to say, finally we've been vindicated. The riots, the putsch, have corroborated our depiction of the crypto-fascist Trump, at last. It's like a twelfth-round knockout or the unmasking of the villain at the end of the final reel. And now with Biden's inauguration today there is palpable relief on the American airwaves. At seventy-eight, Biden is – I learned today – older than Ronald Reagan was when he left office. 'Even allies quietly acknowledge that he is no longer at his prime, meaning he will be constantly watched by friend and foes alike for signs of decline,' quoth the *New York Times*. J Lo, Garth Brooks and Lady Gaga performed.

Twenty-five thousand National Guard troops were in Washington DC to keep the peace. There were fears of a second putsch. But the advertised far-right demonstrators did not materialize. Meanwhile, CNN polls allegedly show that more than thirty per cent of respondents 'did not believe Mr Biden won the election legitimately.' Eighty per cent of Republicans apparently believe this.

Later in the day, word came Biden had signed seventeen executive orders rescinding key parts of the Trump presidency: recommitting the US to the Paris climate accords; overturning the Muslim travel ban.

The Trump era looks like it's consigned to the past. But is it? I have visions of a guerrilla war being waged by far-right insurgents. Maybe now we are in the parallel reality of *Watchmen*, with Biden standing in for Redford. A police force riddled with closet white supremacists and would-be insurrectionists. A little like the South Africa of twenty years ago, with a kind of supersized AWB party resisting the transition to a multicultural multiracial society.

Thursday 21 January

I took Ray to school in the morning. He was crying and complaining about the wind and not wanting to scoot.

'I want to go in the car.'

'We can't go in the car. It's actually against the law.' Which is technically true. There are driving restrictions on the road down to the school.

'It's *too windy*!'

'Let me do up your coat.'

'I DON'T WANT TO.'

'At least put on your gloves.'

'I'M NOT COLD.'

I was despairing. It was one of those moments of utter parental futility when *you* feel like acting like a toddler, lying on the ground screaming and pounding the pavement. In the end, we found a way of travelling he found acceptable, with me cycling alongside him on the pavement and pulling him on his scooter, like a tow truck.

At drop-off I set my bike against a railing, put my mask on and walked up the side of the school playground around the circuitous Covid-safe one-way pedestrian system. Almost no one was around and I felt a little guilty and self-conscious about being judged a key worker. I saw two other children.

'We're late!' Ray said.

'We're not late, we're just in time!'

He became glum again and refused to go into the classroom. The teacher came out to try and help coax him in. She picked up a small branch that was lying on the ground. 'Hey, maybe we can do something with this,' she said. 'Let's take it in.' Ray looked tantalized for a moment. Then lost interest. Finally, with resignation, he went inside.

In the afternoon I recorded a conversation for something called FutureFest – a session that had been delayed nearly a year by Covid and which they'd finally decided to do remotely. I was talking to a music journalist and editor called John Doran. I rambled and did my best impression of a trend spotter and a prognosticator, wanging on about globalism and nativism, prescription drugs and technology and forms of collective madness as a condition of all societies, religions, cultures. I had read up on John beforehand – a talented writer and author of a memoir of extreme alcohol dependency called *Jolly Lad*. Before the chat started I asked him about his book and said to him, 'I've been drinking a lot in lockdown.' 'The thing about alcoholics,' he said, 'is that if you think you might be one, and if you're worrying about drinking too much, you're probably not one. When I was in my most extreme state of addiction, it didn't even occur to me I might have a problem.'

In the evening, I viewed a Joe Exotic cut that was two and a half hours long but showing signs of promise.

Later, I put Ray down. For a few minutes we fired Nerf guns at each other. Then, lying beside each other in his bed, we looked at a lift-the-flap quiz book.

'What is the biggest city in the world? Uh, it's going to be . . . Manila, or Mexico City, or maybe Karachi. Or maybe Tokyo?'

I lifted the flap. *Shanghai*.

'OK, whoops. Next one. What is the brightest star? I think . . . Alpha Centauri.'

I lifted the flap: '*The Sun. During the day.* OK, we knew that. *And at night, Sirius, the dog star.* Zero for two. Try again: The biggest ocean? We've got this: the Pacific.'

'Lift the flap,' Ray said.

'*The Pacific.* Hey! High five!'

At the end there were questions for the reader to answer about themselves.

'Where do you live?' it asked.

Ray said the name of our street. 'In England. In the United Kingdom.'

'Good, Ray-ray. Which languages do you speak?'

'English.'

'What's the weather like today?'

'Windy.'

'And cold and rainy,' I added. 'Where would you most like to explore?'

'Where would you like to explore, Dad?'

'I don't know.' Nowhere was coming to mind. I thought about Scotland and the South of France. Then I said: 'Mexico, maybe. Do you remember we went there? Nice food, friendly people.'

'I want to explore somewhere warm,' Ray said.

'Mexico's pretty warm. OK, time to turn in.'

'Hey, we didn't check the answers,' he said. Seeing my puzzled look, he said, 'Just joking!'

When I tried to leave he clung to me. 'I won't go far, Ray-ray. I'll just be up here working.' I sat with him a little longer and thought about his answers and that he wouldn't have known his street name or probably what country he lives in this time last year. He is getting older. Time is flying by. Life is for living. In the words of Philip Larkin, whether or not you use it, it goes.

Saturday 23 January

I called my mum on FaceTime in the morning. She was at her flat in Eastbourne. She'd been vaccinated a couple of weeks earlier. She'd done it in wholly above-board fashion, but had managed to slip in slightly earlier than others, slipstreaming behind a medical appointment of Michael's, I think, and she was self-conscious that many were still waiting.

Without intending it, as we spoke, I found myself ever so slightly trying to push her buttons.

'I told Nancy's mum about you getting your jab,' I said. 'I tried not to make it sound like you were boasting. She hasn't been vaccinated yet. *She's* waiting until she's called.'

'Well, yes. I used to hate when people told me they'd had the jab and I hadn't. It sounds pushy. I hope it doesn't sound like I've been pushy. Do you think it sounds like I've been pushy?'

'I think that's for you to decide.'

'Well, I don't think I was pushy.'

'Anyway, it sounds like the vaccine isn't so effective against the new variant,' I said.

'I know. I heard that on the radio. But did I tell you about getting it? It was quite a moving experience. There was an atmosphere of calm and it was very well organized. It was in a clinic on Belsize Road and there were volunteers keeping people two metres apart. I think the only thing that would have been better would have been getting it at Salisbury Cathedral. Did you see that?'

'No, I don't think I did.'

'They were in a big line around the cathedral receiving the vaccine. And the organist decided to play music as they did it. It was beautiful.'

'Like a sacrament.'

'Exactly.'

'Remind me, did you have the Pfizer or the BioNTech?'

'I had the AstraZeneca,' my mum said.

'*Dad*, the BioNTech *is* the Pfizer,' Arthur said from across the room. 'The Oxford is the AstraZeneca. They're the same thing.'

'Would you take the Sputnik?' my mum said.

'I don't know. It might have polonium in it.'

Then, remembering the Chinese vaccine, I said: 'What about the Huawei one?'

'Oh yes, I'm not sure about that one.'

'It's got a chip in it and you start feeding bio-data to Alibaba.'

After lunch we went to the local park – me, Jack, Ray, Nancy. Arthur is technically out of self-isolation today. We played a chase game of Ray's devising. 'Someone is infected and they have to infect the other people.'

Sunday 24 January

Around 10.30 it started snowing, the sky filled with flakes and it looked as though it would settle. I FaceTimed my brother.

'Is it snowing where you are?'

'We're on Tooting Common,' he said. 'Look.'

'It just started here.'

'It started here about half an hour ago.'

'It feels healing. It's just what we need.'

'How's that?'

'Magical moment of natural majesty. Nature's bounty bringing us together.'

'I guess,' Marce said, and then: 'Do you find the kids don't really seem that keen on going outside in general?'

'Are you joking? We struggle to keep them *in*. They're always out orienteering and free-soloing up local cliffs. I'm like, "Guys, come in! Get on a screen! *Please*, just for twenty minutes!"'

'Right. "Stop cross-country running and play some Fortnite!"' There was a little pause and he said, 'So Mum said you wangled key worker status.'

'Yes, I did. I work for a public broadcaster, which is one of the categories. Nancy and I both qualified, so we applied and were approved. You understand I didn't give it to myself? We met the criteria.'

'Right,' he said. 'It must be hard up there on the front line facing down the Covid surge.'

'Well, the front line I'm on is in the battle for the nation's morale.'

'Oh, right.'

'You've heard of Dame Vera Lynn? Would you say she was a sort of key worker?'

'Oh, I get it,' he said. 'So *Grounded* is part of the war effort?'

'In a way. I'm keeping up the spirits of a beleaguered nation.'

'But you've got key worker status so you're *not* in fact "grounded",' Marce said.

'Well I *am* grounded. The kids can go to school but I'm locked-down like everyone else. It's not called "My Kids Are Grounded with Louis Theroux". I mean, do you think the nation's morale is important? I don't know. I'm just asking the question. Maybe it isn't. Maybe we just need food and air . . . maybe our souls don't need to be nourished? Is that it? You tell me.'

'OK, Dame Vera, whatever you say.'

After lunch we went out to the park and built a snowman. We made his buttons out of bottle tops and after some debate about names – 'Pebbles', 'Mr Pebble-face' – called him Mr Bottletop. Back at home, we belatedly took down the Christmas tree and decorations, which had been up in a forlorn display for more than a month.

In the news: schools may not reopen until April. Nancy forwarded me an article that said: 'Canadian expert's research finds lockdown harms are 10 times greater than benefits' from the *Toronto Sun*. And the new Brazil and South African variants are present in the UK. Variants are the new front in the war on Covid. The virus is changing and adapting like a monster in a horror film. The most boring horror film ever made.

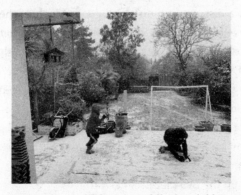

A magical, mood-lifting snowfall, plus children.

Monday 25 January

At two, a man came round with a Covid test. I have to have an up-to-date negative result to be allowed to travel – the Sound-Cloud rap film is moving ahead and there are plans for me to fly to Florida again for the shoot. He appeared at the door, handed me a little packet, and I went upstairs to poke my tonsils and my uvula with a cotton bud. I choked and my eyes watered, then, following the instructions, I snapped off the end of the cotton bud before dropping it into a tiny tube of saline, which I sealed and put into a plastic envelope.

At 3.15, Nancy asked if I'd pick up Ray. 'Just warning you, he'll probably ask to go and see Mr Bottletop.'

I cycled down, riding onto the school grounds since I was running late and there was no one else around. The weather had warmed but the playground still had a thin shell of old snow covering it.

'Can we go and check on Mr Bottletop?' Ray said.

We made our way to the park, me on my bike, Ray on his scooter, arriving at the all-weather sports area where we'd made our snowman. From a distance it didn't look good. Much of the snow was gone, half melted, dirtied. A small group of kids was loitering. One had a long stick of dirty black plastic that he was smashing against the ground where Mr Bottletop had once been. Our arrival had been badly timed to perfection. He was about fourteen years old, pale, not too menacing. Only Mr Bottletop's buttons and two bits of his carrot nose were left. The boy moved away as I approached.

'Were you smashing the snowman?' I asked.

'Nah. It melted,' he said.

I picked up the two pieces of carrot.

'Let's just take his nose, Ray.'

'Sorry,' the boy said. He walked away. 'Better luck next year.'

'I think he did smash it,' Ray said as we left.

'I don't know, Ray. Maybe it did melt. It's not like any of the other snowmen are still around.'

Ray's scooter was on a little leash. He was flagging and I tugged him up the hill and out of one of the park gates, standing aside to let a woman come in with her young son and daughter. I vaguely recognized her, whether from the school gates or just around the local area I couldn't recall.

'All right, Louis?' she said.

'I guess so,' I said.

'How are you coping?'

She had a very slight edge.

'Not brilliant. You know,' I said.

'Yeah. It's shit, isn't it?'

'Yeah. Lockdown. The uncertainty.'

She paused. Then with a meaningful look she said, 'Lockdowns don't work, Louis.'

'Yeah. Well. You should talk to Nancy,' I said.

She raised an eyebrow. 'She works for the BBC, doesn't she?' This was said almost contemptuously. Or at least, with some judgement.

'Not anymore. We started a company together.'

'Oh. Well. OK. I just think the whole thing is wrong and no one is saying anything about it.'

'Well, some people are,' I said.

'Why don't *you* say something about it?'

I felt put on the spot. 'Social media,' I said. 'It's so polarizing. I don't know what to say. Just to offer an opinion, you're making yourself a lightning rod for all the hate.'

'My husband's a consultant. So he goes to school.' She gestured at her five-year-old. 'So we have it fairly easy. People don't understand what a lot of us are going through. I used to be left-wing but it's the right-wingers I agree with now.'

'It's very hard,' I said. 'I wish I had some answers.'

Back at the house, I worked for a bit. Ray was on the iPad. At five I stopped. Ray and Nancy had built a fort on his bed out of cushions and blankets and we climbed into that and pretended to sleep and then pretended to have breakfast.

Downstairs, I made dinner and listened to the radio – Evan Davis on Radio 4. There was a dark feeling of brewing mutiny, people chafing at the restrictions. *The mental health of children is suffering*, they were saying. *Homeschoolers can't cope.*

I thought about homeschoolers not coping. I thought about weird feelings of anger, of being fed up. School children going slowly insane . . . it was building up. The need to lash out and blame and the resentment at being told what to do, being lied to, and nothing getting better. It felt bad.

Ray's school has been telling them about 'ow-ows' on the inside. They colour code them: red is for angry; blue is for sad.

Can you imagine anything more divisive – more diabolical, in a way? A virus that preys on the weak and the elderly. Shaving the margins – nudging the herd to turn upon those who are already slow and vulnerable. And the only measures that may help will constrain and sacrifice life in general – punish the young, the vigorous, anyone in the entire rest of the world who isn't old and infirm. As if to put people to the test and ask: *You say you value life, but at what cost to the young?*

I am supposed to be flying on Sunday but now there's some doubt as to whether I can go – possible new rules about needing to quarantine in a hotel for ten days when I get back. Which would make it impossible.

Tuesday 26 January

Milestone of 100,000 deaths in the UK. Two million deaths worldwide. Increase in cases accelerating. There are signs of new infections slowing in America but they haven't been hit by the UK variant yet. No one really knows what's happening next.

We are fraying at the edges here. Tetchy and short-tempered. Seeing their friends less, going out less, seems to make the kids want to see their friends less and go out less. Anxiety and upset in an awful feedback loop. A horrendous shouting match today with Jack, to do with a friend who was coming over to go on the half-pipe in a neighbour's garden. Jack said it was covered in snow and ice.

'So sweep it!' I said.

'YOU SWEEP IT!' he shouted.

From the older kids I have the impression I am an irritant, or at best an irrelevance. 'No one asked you. Flip off. Idiot.' Today, after receiving a heap of abuse, I said to Nancy, 'I don't know what to do. I need advice. My child is telling me to shut up.' I was angrier than I realized – I actually thought I was calm – and I strolled over and snatched the phone out of Jack's hand.

He looked shocked for a moment, and then regarded me with disdain. 'At least be polite about it,' he said, and walked out.

'What are you *doing*?' Nancy said. 'You didn't give him any warning.'

'I don't know! I don't know what I'm doing! I said I need advice.'

I plugged in the phone to charge, then felt ashamed at having snatched it and thought about giving it back, then I thought: *When you're in a hole, stop digging. Just leave it.* But a bout of shame and despair and self-doubt followed, disbelief at my own failings as a parent. I never expected to be so bad at this, running around, throwing tantrums over trivial arguments, getting into fights with my children.

We are struggling. It is hard. It is very hard.

The *New York Times* today said: 'CDC officials say most available evidence indicates schools can be safe if precautions are taken on campus and in the community.'

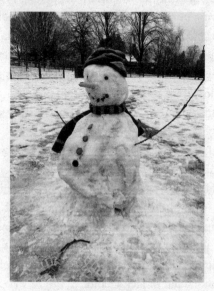

Mr Bottletop.

Thursday 28 January

And so life goes on with no end in sight. Covid will be around for years . . . I suppose we knew that . . . and it's a matter of living with it . . . The expert on the radio today said she didn't want to speculate but used the word 'years'. Not much leisure travel likely in 2021, says the *Today* programme. The roll-out of the vaccine is imperative because the more the virus spreads, the more likely a variant arises that is vaccine-resistant.

This evening, at supper, as a bit of macabre humour, I said, 'This could be our dinosaur moment.'

'I don't think so, Dad,' Jack said. 'If it couldn't kill Michael Rosen, I don't think it'll wipe out our entire species.'

But it does feel as though this is the spur to humility we perhaps needed, a glimpse of the insecurity of our tenancy on Planet Earth. We imagined ourselves the apex predators, and felt appropriately guilty, but here we are made hostages, not of Godzilla, or an invading alien, or hyper-intelligent apes, or killer bees, but a life force so basic it's not even clear whether it is a life form. A virus. A self-replicating scrap of DNA wrapped in protein. Imagine. If we are wiped out by Covid, maybe in ten million years the virus will evolve into an intelligent life form: crown-shaped virus-people in virus-cities, listening to virus-SoundCloud rap and going to virus-far-right rallies.

Earlier in the day we'd had the usual melodrama of rage and hysteria, moments of grumpiness and comedy and the hypomania that is children and parents grappling with their mental health, when they can't get out much, they can't see people, and the end seems very far away, if it is an end. Shouting about whether children were doing their classes. Ray not wanting his 'Jelly and Josh' YouTube show to end. At parents' evening with Jack's teachers, a succession of kindly faces on our computer said versions of, 'He is enormously able and has always been a pleasure to have in class but he has not been turning up for many of his Google Classroom lessons or uploading his assignments.'

I had a low-level feeling of sadness and guilt and an urge to bail on my trip to America on Sunday. I'm fifty – do I need to be chasing SoundCloud rappers and alt-righters around Florida? Glugging sizzurp and marching on the Capitol in a bicycle helmet, so I can scoop up garlands at awards ceremonies, while my children go under-parented, failing to turn up for their Google Classroom and getting older without me being around.

It makes me think, maybe for the first time, of maybe taking a different path. Being behind the scenes. *Just being more at home.*

When I went in to kiss Jack goodnight he said, 'Why were you so disappointed with what the teachers said?'

'Because you're capable of so much more, Jack. You have a great mind. And it's not just about doing well at school, it's about you feeling connected to something and being proud of doing your best.'

Then we hugged.

Friday 29 January

News full of Redditors who shook the markets in defence of GameStop – an American electronics goods chain – where, as it happens, I bought my first Google Home smart speaker at its West Hollywood branch in 2017.

The company is like RadioShack or Currys: a down-on-its-luck old-school bricks-and-mortar retail chain. Hedge fund investors were shorting the GameStop stock, making money off its declining prospects. But the online community decided to come to its rescue en masse, using populist online trading platforms to invest, driving up the GameStop stock price, and costing various hedge fund fat cats hundreds of millions.

One of the open-to-anyone trading portals, Robinhood, closed its doors to random traders, evidently feeling that the disruption had gone too far, then politicos waded in, with an unlikely populist alliance between arch right-winger Ted Cruz and leftie Alexandra Ocasio-Cortez, both of whom saw something to like in the idea of mass participation in the markets shaking up the elites

Arthur said, 'All my For You page says is stuff about GameStop.'

'What is a "For You page"?' I asked.

'Never mind,' he said.

I don't know if it means anything, except that it feels the perfect expression of 2021 insurgency, and there is satisfaction in 'business as usual' being discomfited. The world's richest man, Elon Musk, is on the side of the populist insurgents, tweeting 'Get Shorty!', which may be all you need to know.

In the afternoon, I dragged Ray off his iPad. 'We're going out, OK? Time to get some fresh air.'

'Where are we going?' Ray asked.

I mentioned the three local parks, then said: 'Or we could go somewhere a little scary. There are a lot of dead people there.'

'Where?'

'Kensal Green Cemetery.'

'What's a cemetery?'

'A graveyard. It's where they put the dead people.'

Arthur agreed to come too. We made the short drive. 'Ooh! Spooky cemetery gates,' Arthur said as we arrived, playing along.

We were at the upper end of the cemetery, near the Catholic area, close to Scrubs Lane. It had been raining for much of the day and there were puddles along the path. I'd brought a couple of frisbees and a football. Ray was enjoying kicking the ball into puddles then trying to a lasso it out with a bungee cord he'd found in the back of the car.

I pressed on, a little ahead, enjoying the vista of the large open space filled with monuments, headstones and tiny crosses squashed next to each other, disordered like a supersized version of the bric-a-brac you might find on a mantlepiece: the venerable, the austere alongside the kitsch.

I heard a cry. Ray was in tears, pointing at his trousers, which were soaked down one side with muddy water. He'd fallen into a puddle. Arthur offered to wipe him down and I gave him my scarf.

'It doesn't feel nice,' he wailed. 'I want to go somewhere else.'

I picked him up. 'We could play hide and seek?'

This placated him and we made our way further into the cemetery, finding our path blocked by larger and larger puddles. Whole areas of the cemetery were submerged in temporary ponds, and we had to make our way over the grass to find a way through. Most of the trees were leafless and twisted, but there were also yews with their needles on and ivy and other evergreens. The grass was uneven, the grave plots tilted and ramshackle. We were at the southernmost edge and could look down at the Grand Union Canal and in the distance see building works, a new apartment block on the A40. Ray was shouting, happy now, and I noticed a mourner standing in silent contemplation, seemingly in tears. 'Hey, Ray-ray, try to keep it down,' I said.

We were in an area where the graves were smaller, and some had small toys on them. I read a headstone and realized we were in the children's cemetery. There were headstones for babies and toddlers. Some had photos and epitaphs that bore references to them being 'born sleeping' and seeing them again one day.

'This is where they bury the babies that died, Ray,' I said. Then, seeing a serried rank of small rectangular stones, in perfect formation. 'And over there is where they buried the soldiers after the First World War.'

'Is that where the king is buried?' Ray asked, pointing at a larger monument.

'No, I don't think so.'

'Where did they bury the king?'

'I think they buried the kings at Windsor maybe, in the royal family chapel.'

We made our way back down to a central pathway. Arthur was looking for an old grave. 'This one is 1903, Dad.'

'Most of the older ones are on the other side. Some go back to the 1830s.'

Ray was growing impatient. 'When are we going to play hide and seek?' I was trying to find a spot that was a little open and away from the central track, which cars were using. Ray, losing patience, said, 'I want to go somewhere else, Dad!'

'Shall we just go home?'

'I don't want to go home!'

Arthur pretended to be a zombie, and chased Ray, briefly lifting his mood. 'What about hide and seek?'

'OK, let's do it here.' We were at a monument that had been

fashioned like a very large gazebo, with three or four park benches. One of the benches had a lifelike bronze figure of the deceased man. The monument was pristine; it looked new, and there was Arabic text inscribed around it. There were fresh plants and flowers, a pair of vigorous looking olive trees in tubs. There was also what appeared to be a real football at the man's feet and a real woollen football supporter's scarf around his neck. Behind one of the benches were cleaning implements – a bucket, a broom, a mop.

Ray was stroking the bronze man's knee. 'Can I hug him?'

'I guess. If you want to. OK, you count first.'

We played three rounds, one person seeking, the others hiding and trying to reach a bench next to the monument.

As we ran and laughed and chased, under the gaze of the bronze seated man, I couldn't figure out whether we were showing insufficient reverence, or maybe doing him the honour of including him in the ongoing pleasures of the still-living.

'One more round, Ray.'

Arthur was losing patience. 'I thought we were doing three.'

'I know but it's kind of fun.'

Afterwards, we trudged back. Ray's mood dipped again. 'That was fun, wasn't it?' I said.

'I hated it,' Ray said. 'It was the worst day of my life.'

Sunday 31 January

Rushing around the house to get ready to fly – trimming my beard, trying to help with kids. Feeling sad.

'I wish I wasn't going,' I said to Nancy.

'You've got to make programmes. Other people are putting the work in.'

As I packed, downstairs, I heard shouting. Jack.

'He wanted to go straight out to the games room,' Nancy said. 'No breakfast, not changed.'

'You need to do some homework, Jack.'

'It's the weekend!'

'Yes, it's the weekend. That's when you do homework. At the weekend. When you're *at home*.'

Nancy: 'You're going to on-site school on Monday. I can't have this! Daddy is going away and I have work to do.'

In the end, after a lot of shouting, he went upstairs and did one of his assignments. Then went on the PlayStation.

At 10.15 my taxi arrived. I'd got most of the things done I needed to. Except my hair. With salons and barbers all closed, I haven't had a trim for months. Nancy was supposed to give me a haircut and that never happened.

Exhausted, on the way to the airport, I fell into a grateful sleep.

February 2021

SOUNDCLOUD

Friday 5 February

Florida

So, here we are. More than a year on from when we actively began the research into SoundCloud rap, nearly four years on from my first impulse to make a programme about the subject, we've finally embarked on a *wholly new project*, and the not-so-good news is that the scene appears to be deceased. Yes, I know, it's a shame we didn't figure that out before we flew, but I guess I was distracted by other things. The truth is, even a year ago, pre-Covid, we might have struggled. The world of emo rap music, uploaded onto the platform SoundCloud from which it takes its name, in which cartoonish MCs with brightly coloured hair and facial tattoos spit lyrics of aggressive stupidity like 'Gucci Gang Gucci Gang Gucci Gang Gucci Gang Gucci Gang Gucci Gang' was probably on its uppers even then. The death of Juice WRLD, on the back of the deaths of Lil Peep and XXXTentacion, was maybe the last gasp. Have I lost the attention of the general non-rap-listening audience yet?

You get the feeling now that asking people about 'SoundCloud' is a little embarrassing, like asking them about the Osmonds or Acid Jazz.

The first few days we made studio visits with a couple of guys who I had the feeling were big maybe a year or three ago – nice people, one called BamSavage, another named OnStar Cruz – neither of them, I think, in any danger of troubling the upper reaches of the charts anytime soon. Our closest thing to a prospect was a tiny Cuban kid called BrokeBaby, who looks almost Dickensian in the sense of ill health he gives off. With his inked-up cheeks and vaunted opiate use, he could be a SoundCloud poster boy, and in fact in the year since we first met him, he has lost his best friend and fellow rapper Mikey Swah to a heroin overdose. Mikey, memorably, had 'Fuck You' tattooed on his eyelids.

BrokeBaby's videos show him waving guns and boasting about chucking back prescription drugs, Xanax and Percocets. In his social media clips, he snorts lines of cocaine. 'Ignorant shit' sells, he said. Provocation gets traction on social media. It doesn't even have to be real. 'Fake it till you make it.' But Broke – no disrespect to him – I suspect doesn't represent the future of the genre. He has never matched the numbers of his debut record 'PunkBaby' (sample lyric: 'Bitch I'm on shit / Pop a Percocet'). Two days running, a video shoot we were supposed to film him at failed to materialize.

It's a weird feeling being on a shoot that's showing signs of being a washout. The worst of it is the hanging around, the hours passing at the hotel, though at least on this occasion I've been keeping busy working on other stuff, watching cuts of the Joe Exotic doc, feeding back notes, conference calls on other projects. We had been hoping that we might get the whole film in the can in one trip. In hindsight that was ridiculously over-optimistic. We'll be lucky to get half and from time to time I have found myself wondering if there is a story here at all. There is also the awareness that this is a Mindhouse production: the company coffers are being depleted paying for hotels and crew while we sit here and accomplish very little.

Not helping is a sense of civilizational collapse on the home front. Me being away is a strain on Nancy at the best of times, but with the kids in lockdown that is even more the case. She is a lone hold-out on a frontier where the barbarians are revolting. This may be her Teutoburg Forest.

On Thursday, Jack turned thirteen. The first time I can recall that I've been away for one of the boys' birthdays. I called home in the morning and all seemed well. Nancy had taken time off work and Jack had opened his presents. I'd recorded a video message, sending love and hugs. I'd found an old video from when he was three years old or so, in his underpants, and doing a dance as I filmed on my phone. 'What are you doing?' I'd asked.

'It's called a boomy dance,' he'd said.

For my message I showed a little clip of the boomy dance, and then I sent a text that said, **Have a boomy dance day!**

In the morning, Jack's reply: **Thanks, Dad, love you Xx.** And then: **Maybe it's the end of the boomy dance era but you never know.**

Later in the day I called again – en route to a studio where we were meeting rappers and producers. There was a funny mood in the house. Jack seemed forlorn.

'Arthur and Ray are *not* behaving well,' Nancy said. 'Ray has gone full-on Kevin. So poor Jack hasn't been having a good birthday.'

Later she rang again.

Nancy: 'Ray went crazy.'

Me: 'But he's done that before. Tipping over chairs and chucking his toys around.'

Nancy: 'Yes, but this lasted two hours and he was screaming.'

Me: 'What did he want?'

Nancy: 'He wanted to play "it".'

Me: 'Oh wow, I'm sorry. Yeah, it's been tricky here too. Cuts to watch. Trying to stay on top of the shoot. I'm spinning so many plates it's insane.'

Nancy: 'What did you say?'

Me: 'I know you're spinning plates too.'

Nancy: 'You have no idea.' She raised a middle finger to the screen.

Me: 'Nancy, don't do that. You're giving me blue ow-ows on the inside. I've got plates I'm spinning too. Why can't we both be spinning plates?'

Nancy: 'You said it was *insane*. You're there with your coffee brewing on your desk and people making meals for you.'

Me: 'OK. Fair enough. It's not insane.'

I blame myself in some ways for the production doldrums: for not being more engaged before we left. For being distracted during our pre-trip Zoom call. Also, because I've been watching Joe Exotic cuts and recording voice-over from the hotel, I've not been putting my shoulder to the wheel the way I might have – making calls and trawling the Internet and driving the research and galvanizing the team. Team galvanization has never been my strong suit.

Anyway, as I write this, it finally feels like we are making a little headway on our story. Tonight, we met a rapper called Ratchet Roach, a friendly giant with dreads and tattoos on his face, who keeps a pistol in his waistband. He used to be tight with XXX-Tentacion and while he's never had a big hit in his own right he embodies the old-school values of the street code, with an approach to the criminal lifestyle that carries its own kind of integrity. He gives off a restrained menace that is in its way charming. So from thinking the shoot might be a bust, there are now signs of life, if we forget the idea of 'SoundCloud' and look at it as being more generally about crime and rap music in Florida.

Saturday 6 February

Drove four and a half hours to Tampa for an outdoor car and rap show at the Florida State Fairgrounds. Spread out over several acres under the hot Florida sun, with car sound systems blaring and generators roaring, it was a cacophonous headache-inducing heatscape. We were chaperoned around by Miss Kia, the editor of a rap magazine called *My Hood*. She introduced us to the event organizer, a man in a blue T-shirt called DawgMan.

Midday I sat in the crew vehicle and told Ray a bedtime story via FaceTime, about looking for buried treasure with his friend Artie, and running into a pirate called Pirate Pete. Then the performances started and I interviewed a parade of aspiring artists from around the country as they prepared to go on stage. They had names like Lord Menace and Roxxanne Montana and Lil Polo Don. Alas, due to losing my iPhone, we arrived too late to speak to Money Bagg Yo. The headliner was a hot act from Memphis called Pooh Shiesty. He's only twenty or so, was signed by Atlanta trap legend Gucci Mane, and raps with an infectious southern drawl. His hottest record, 'Back in Blood', is a cheeky flex about his supposed habit of robbing people without wearing a mask, with an invitation for them to come and try to get their stuff, if they think they're up to it. I'm paraphrasing.

(Incidentally, the not-wearing-masks part is not a point about not observing Covid protocols, but a suggestion that he is so unworried about retribution that he has no need to conceal his identity. Just to clear that up.)

There was a mounting sense of anxiety from DawgMan as it seemed likely that Pooh might be late for his advertised slot of 8 p.m. and might not show at all. In the end, he arrived around 8.30, emerged from his blacked-out tour van trailing a retinue of fans and associates, then went onstage for a set that lasted a little under ten minutes and consisted of him rapping over a backing track in a big huddle of hangers-on, of whom I was one, stage extreme right, and then retreating back to the tour van, as fans and local rappers took turns to be allowed inside to take photos with Pooh for $100 each.

We had previously made contact with Pooh Shiesty's manager, Big Boy, and the possibility of an interview had been floated. Feeling self-conscious amid the entourage loitering by the van door, I said loudly, 'Interview with the BBC? BBC documentary?'

Finally, at around 10 p.m., tired and a little nervous, I was ushered in, and took up a seat on a vinyl banquette at the back, our knees touching, the air full of smoke – me wondering if it was all Covid safe. He had a large oil painting of himself, given to him by a fan, propped up next to him, and from time to time he would offer it a puff on his blunt.

I was aware how limited my time was and went at the interview with puppyish eagerness, notwithstanding that I'd been flayed and pummelled by ten-plus hours of cacophonous clashing sound systems and hot sun and a battery of shouty vox-pop-style interviews with up-and-comers. Pooh batted away questions about his recent criminal issues – he was out on bond for $60,000 having been charged with shooting, though not killing, two young men who thought they were meeting up with him to sell him some weed and some expensive shoes. I asked him about his case – what would he like to say about it? He paused, peered through a wreath of blunt smoke and said, simply, 'It's Shiesty Season.' A great example of the media strategy: If you don't like the question you've been asked, then answer something else. In this case, *What is the name of your new album?*

Twenty or so minutes in, Pooh's manager gave us the wind-it-up sign and we tumbled off the bus, dazed but with the feeling of at least having something to show for all the hours of waiting.

We went to a VIP after party, for some nightlife shots, having been invited along by DawgMan and hoping to maybe cement some relationships with Pooh and other stars. No VIPs were in evidence, it was more of a semi-socially distanced sort-of-outside in tents shindig for people who'd presumably paid an extra fifty dollars. I drank cocktails at the bar, as the flashy and fabulous partygoers lounged and listened to a pair of excitable DJs who spun Mark Morrison's 'Return of the Mack' – the Midlands-raised nineties R&B singer is enjoying an unlikely renaissance in Central Florida. I reflected how strange it was to be clubbing and drinking while everyone I knew back home was locked down. Filming-wise, it wasn't getting us much but I was having a surreal old-school non-Covid nightclub experience, necking gin and tonics in the middle of the pandemic. At midnight we called it and drove back to Miami, arriving around 5 a.m. The hotel had no record of my reservation, and a slow-moving receptionist called Wes Chang tried to sort it out. Upstairs I took my mind off the long day by reading Kazuo Ishiguro's novel *The Buried Giant* for fifteen minutes.

Friday 12 February

Florida

More frustration, followed by a small breakthrough. A four-hour trip back to Tampa, from Miami, on Sunday, based on a call from Pooh's manager and invitation to the studio, went suddenly cold, texts unreturned. We cooled our heels at Starbucks, stared disconsolately at our phones, did laundry at the hotel, then, the following day, a depressing drive back to Miami. Then, at the evening shoot in a high crime area of Pompano Beach with Ratchet Roach, a kind of hood orientation that felt like maybe it was a helpful scene, though they were playing up the danger of the area so much I wondered if I was being patronized. I had the unwelcome image of myself as a *Blue Peter* presenter, explaining to children, 'And it's very exciting because this is one of the most crime-plagued areas of greater Miami, and Ratchet's agreed to show us around.' I was also aware that the story was just clinging on to life. Then, another small lead, to a twenty-two-year-old music video director and mini-mogul, with diamond grills on his teeth and £1,300 shoes, who goes by the professional moniker DrewFilmedIt. Drew had offered to introduce us to an Orlando rapper he works with called Hotboii – his latest track, 'Don't Need Time', a plaintive paean to a dead homey, has 45 million views on YouTube and has just gone gold, whatever that means in an era when no one buys records.

With Drew, we drove round to a plush studio in a quiet residential neighbourhood. The house had high brick walls around it, almost like it was designed to repel bullets. Hotboii has been involved in a feud with another Orlando rapper named 9lokknine – allegedly there have been several shootings because of the beef – and I had the impression that Drew was twitchy, spooked in a more than ordinary way by a passing car or chopper in the sky.

When we arrived, Hotboii was in a mixing booth listening to a playback. He is twenty and has four thick dreadlocks that point up a foot or more up in the air and are tied together at the top like a frame for runner beans. We went out to a patio and he rolled a big blunt and answered questions about his upbringing, his mum struggling to provide for him and his four siblings, how he resorted to robbing iPhones and burgling houses to provide for himself. We talked for an hour or so. He was open on almost every topic I brought up – his preferred drugs (weed rather than drank), the problem of 'clout chasing' (up-and-comers resorting to low tactics like picking fights in order to build their followings). He even chuckled when I asked him about his alleged feud with 9lokknine. Alas, I may have been undone by hubris. Something unsettled him – possibly a question about social media – and his face clouded over. 'These questions be retarded,' he said, and picked up his bag and walked off. Normally a walk-off is a useful moment of conflict in a film, but here it was so unexpected, and also so counter to the flow of the conversation, which was warm and forthcoming, that I don't imagine we'll use it. And so I felt bad about ending on a wrinkle of misunderstanding, and I apologized to Drew and to Hotboii's manager, but mainly I was relieved to have filmed something solid for the documentary.

Anyway, here we are. We were out here two weeks, we still have a way to go, but we have made a start. What's been difficult is being conscious of burning up goodwill with Nancy, as she struggles at home, working full time, helping to run the company, the kids growing crazed, cooped-up, locked-down, homeschooling, and every second taking a toll on the relationship. Her upset, her wanting so much to support me, stressed about work, about the kids and them not engaging with their remote learning, cleaning, cooking, laundry, everything on top of her.

'It's impossible,' she said, in tears. 'I can't do it. It's impossible.'

'I know, Nancy. It's hard enough with two of us, so to do it on your own . . .'

I also think back to last March. Back then we were about to shoot SoundCloud rap. We had no idea what was coming. Climbing back into production feels a little like getting up to dance after being too-long seated, joints and legs stiff, nothing moving quite right. And I also know it might have been every bit as hard then. Worlds like rap and hip hop, where there is both star power and an endemic level of suspicion of outsiders, can be hard to crack at any time. The culture has moved on, the scene is different, but it is also very much the same. Crime, money, social media. 'Vaunting aloud, but racked with deep despair.' Milton's line about Satan in *Paradise Lost* also applies to a lot of rappers.

In news from the UK, meanwhile, word comes that the R rate is below one for the first time since July. On 22 February, Boris Johnson will unveil a 'roadmap to the easing of lockdown.' Schools may reopen on 8 March. So in the darkest times there is what seems to be the glimmer of dawn. Or maybe just the latest step in a year-long hokey-cokey dance of restrictions being lifted and then reimposed. 'Widespread easing likely by May,' says the news. But some scientists are saying restrictions must remain. Does it feel like the end of the pandemic is on the horizon? No.

Still, it feels like we are close to the end of something. Not the end of the measures or the end of the pandemic. But maybe the end of me being interested in the pandemic?

Saturday 13 February

I arrived home just after midday. I had upgraded myself to business on the plane, paying $700 or $800 out of my own pocket for the luxury of a few hours on a flat bed.

I loved being back and made a point of saying to Nancy several times, 'I'm so happy to be back,' which I was.

After supper I took Ray up and told him the latest instalment of the long-running Pirate Pete story, which involved aliens and an evil shipmate called Cutlass Chris and another very silly shipmate called Ridickleeous Ronnie who kept pooing his pants. I was so tired I nodded off as I was speaking and awoke to hear myself in a half-dream state uttering the nonsense phrase, 'retrofitted T-shirts'.

'Sorry, Ray, I dropped off,' I said, and resumed the story.

Sunday 14 February

Arthur's birthday. Presents in the morning. I'd also bought bonus gifts for the other boys, due to me being away for Jack's birthday on the fourth and due to Ray being only six years old. Toblerone mini-candies and a *Korea for Geeks* book for Jack and a Ravensburger space puzzle and a board game called Frustration for Ray.

We played Frustration, me and Nancy and Ray and Art. Ray, after having his men sent back to base several times, fell into a funk, feeling *overly* frustrated. He began trying to sneak his men out, then, on his turn, would repeatedly roll his dice until he got a six. Afterwards, he said: 'I don't like my present,' and then began shouting, over and over again, 'I want more presents.'

'It's not your birthday, Ray. You can't have more presents.'

'I WANT MORE PRESENTS!'

'This is what he was like on Jack's birthday,' Nancy said. 'Except it lasted an hour and a half. *I want to play "it"*.'

Then angst from upstairs because Arthur's sea-spray hair spritzer didn't give his hair the adequate sea-sprayed quality.

My mum and Michael came by in masks. In the end they came inside and had coffees.

'Yes, I enjoyed your conversation with Justin,' my mum said. I'd interviewed my cousin, the actor and filmmaker Justin Theroux, for *Grounded*. 'It was entertaining. But I thought you were a bit rude about Melvyn Bragg. And I thought you were a bit down on your Westminster education.'

'The Bragg thing was affectionate, really,' I said. 'And as for school, that was me making the point that Justin had struggled in a mainstream educational setting but had gone on to great success.'

'Well, yes,' my mum said.

I couldn't, for some reason, let it lie, and had another go, warming to my theme a little too much. 'Latin and rote learning, the stuff they teach at Westminster, it's cobblers,' I went on. 'It's just crammer stuff. Memorization, becoming a drone . . . Justin's won two Emmies. He's a beloved screenwriter and director.'

'I wouldn't say it was cobblers,' my mum said.

In the afternoon, we went to Hyde Park and walked around the Serpentine. I was bleary with jet lag but Nancy was full of beans, racing Ray and lifting chunks of ice out of the water and kicking them around the bank. I'd brought a plastic Ziploc bag of brussels sprouts leftovers from the freezer for the ducks and geese. They were not a hit. When we got back the boys got on their devices and I nodded off in a chair.

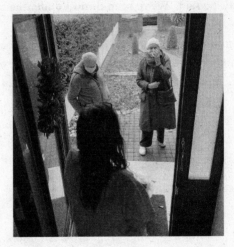

A doorstep visit from my mum and Michael.

Monday 15 February

Half-term

I was up at seven to watch a cut of episode two of our snooker series. It looked good, close to being excellent. A feeling of pride in having been a small part of birthing a non-me-fronted project. This was always the dream, and it's happening. Mindhouse. Even the name, with the patina of a year's use, now has an antique gravity to it.

After Ray drop-off I bumped into a guy who owns several gastropubs.

'Hospitality,' he said. 'We've been thrown under the bus.'

I told him about being an essential worker.

'Yeah, me too. I changed my pubs into delis so I qualified. Still, school fees are six-thousand a year so I had a bit of leverage. Let's face it, the Filipino at the house wasn't going to do the home schooling.'

Tuesday 16 February

I awoke this morning still half in dreamworld. I've been jet-lagged, not sleeping enough or well when I do sleep. I got up feeling half drowned, soggy with a tiredness that was soaked into my muscle and my bones and around my eyes. Downstairs, I did a little bit of a puzzle with Ray before he jumped on the iPad.

In the afternoon, I dragged Ray and Jack out to the park. At the playground I pushed them on the big round swing. Then Ray wanted to play a game he calls 'levels', that involves me setting him tasks: 'Climb up the slide in your socks and then slide back down.' It requires quite a bit of resourcefulness to keep thinking of missions, given you're working with a couple of small climbing frames, some logs, and that's about it.

Ray: 'Dad, what level am I on?'

Me: 'Level 2,031.'

Ray: 'What do I have to do to get to the next level?'

Me: 'Balance across all these logs.'

Ray: 'What? We already did that.'

Me: 'Right, but now you have to do it while clapping your hands.'

Wednesday 17 February

Rain all day. I did not at any point leave the house, unless taking out the recycling counts.

Thursday 18 February

Half-decent weather. The sun has been out. The sky was clear and bright. In the afternoon it was verging on spring-like and I felt an almost ineffable lifting of the mood and a sense of hope. The world came into sharper focus as a place promising a future. Nancy took the kids out to the park while I made calls.

In the evening, Nancy said, to someone on the phone, 'That's great news. He'll be really pleased.'

Off the phone, she said, 'Joe Wicks commission.'

It has been gestating for months. My lockdown guru and inspiration, Mr Spider-Man Lunges himself, the man who has been keeping me sane – alongside a carefully calibrated regimen of alcohol-based decoctions – will be part of the Mindhouse family. A single documentary looking at family and mental health and getting back on track as we come out of lockdown. It's been through various iterations as it's gone back and forth to the channel commissioners as a two-parter, a three-parter, something formatted around a school or a council estate, in a Gareth Malone kind of way, or in a *Jamie's School Dinners* kind of way.

In the end it became something simpler and deeper, a look at Joe's work through its origin story in his family life and upbringing. I'd heard him on *Desert Island Discs*, and his account of growing up with parents both of whom were affected by mental illness – dad heroin dependent, mum OCD – was extraordinarily moving, all the more so for the aura of perfection Joe projects, with his immaculate home and his luxuriant hair. So the documentary will interweave a revisit to Joe's past with a look at other families grappling with mental health as we emerge from Covid. It will be more than a project for me. It will be part of a mission. The mission to get people moving. I know I sound like a brainwashed groupie, but I am a believer.

I congratulated Nancy on the commission – it was her work, alongside her team – that had made it happen. We'd finished supper and for a while we sat in companionable silence. The good news, and maybe the soft sunlight, conspired to create a moment. I thought about how lucky I was to have Nancy, and I thought back over the previous months, and the strange discovery, which shouldn't have been surprising, of how much I enjoyed working with her, and how talented she was, how driven, and how committed to our work, and should we have done this years earlier? Or had I needed time to gain confidence, or to find the right team to work alongside us, like Arron and Sophie? But in any case, we were here now, in the unlikely and, if I was honest, never-truly-envisioned-on-my-part position of having the beginnings of a successful TV company.

Then, I said, 'Why did you disconnect from me?'

'A really big thing for me . . .' she said.

'What?'

'Your drinking. It was like you would check out.'

'I hardly drank in America. Couple of beers at night. If that.'

'Why were you drinking so much?' she said.

'Don't know. Anxiety? Boredom?' I was thinking: *Because I enjoyed it.* 'Do you want to sit on my lap?' I said.

'With the kids around?' They were on their phones.

She sat on my lap and I kissed her and told her I loved her.

'Ooh cringe. Can you stop?' Jack said.

Friday 19 February

At bedtime, Ray said, 'The coronavirus is nearly over, right, Dad?'

'I'm not sure. I hope so. What makes you say that?'

'Because it's been here a year.'

'Well, not quite a year. Though I suppose it has. In fact, you're right.'

We lay down together and told a continuation of the nightly story but got lost in where we were. I improvised a plot to do with treasure in our local park and the coronavirus – one of the baddies had been going around spraying it on car door handles – and a burglar that stole jewellery from next door. He turned out to be Pirate Pete in disguise. Afterwards, Nancy and I had a long drunken intercontinental Zoom drinks party with friends in London, Weymouth and Toronto. I chucked back the tequila and we told jokes and caught up. None of my repartee was landing. I realized we weren't being heard very clearly and got my podcast microphone. After that, everything went more smoothly.

Saturday 20 February

More mild weather. Glimmers of hope but an equivocal hope that still involves masks and anxiety.

Sunday 21 February

The sun was out. We drove to Windsor Great Park, a vast royal park of rhododendron forests and huge conifers, sequoias, redwoods, in stately grounds forty-five minutes' drive out of London. We had brought a picnic from Gail's Bakery and also a polystyrene toy glider which I'd ordered online. We made our way into the park, past other walkers, along a well-trodden path.

'Can we please go this way?' Jack said, gesturing into the groves of rhododendrons, which had one or two gaps that might lead to tracks.

'We're looking for somewhere to stop and eat. Those tracks don't go anywhere.'

'This path is so dead!' Jack said. 'You guys are literally *spamming out the park*.'

'What does that even mean?' I said.

No answer.

'Art, do you know what that means?'

He couldn't resist a smile. 'He's using gamer speak. It just means overusing it.'

We found some open ground with a log that was used as a bench and broke out our picnic from the backpacks. Then we got out the glider, had a few throws. Jack took over and on his first throw managed to land it halfway up a conifer.

'I knew this would happen,' Nancy said.

'Can you climb it?'

Jack climbed the interior of the branches and Nancy found a long stick. A combination of shaking and nudging dislodged the plane. A few more throws. Jack and Ray romped after the plane to be the one to throw next.

'Guys, just take turns!' Nancy said. But the chase was hard to resist, and within a minute or two, Ray, trying to outrun Jack and reach the plane first, collapsed on top of it, breaking the wing.

'I knew it!' Nancy said.

The wing wasn't completely off. Jack threw it again. 'It's fine, look!' The plane, listing badly, managed a short flight. 'See, it's not even broken.'

'Don't waggle it!'

I picked it up and bent the wing slightly. It was 90 per cent gone. I threw it: It flew again but even worse.

'Dad broke it!'

'Jack! Seriously?'

'Dad broke it and he's trying to blame me.'

Ray was crying.

'I can glue it,' I said. 'It'll be like new.'

'I want a new one,' Ray said.

'Fine, we can get a new one.'

'I want two new ones.'

Vaccinations are rolling out – 17 million have had at least one jab. Allegedly the R number is going down. But hospitalizations, at more than 17,500, aren't far off what they were at the height of Lockdown One.

Latest daily figure for deaths in the UK: 215.

Monday 22 February

Announcement from Johnson today at 7 p.m.: all schools back by 8 March. Teachers' unions not happy. Friends can meet in parks in small numbers and six people can get together in a garden outside, or two families if that's bigger. It's all a bit confusing and nonsensical but the signal is that we can relax a tiny bit. Numbers trending down.

At supper, I said, 'That's the last of the lockdowns, I reckon. Whatever happens next.'

'Dad, you literally said that last lockdown,' Jack said.

March 2021

TROLLS

Monday 1 March

I don't even know if it needs explanation *why* I'd decided I needed to make a programme about the new underground of far-right Trump-supporting Internet trolls. If you've followed my work, you'll know I've done stories on white nationalists of different stripes many times over the years. The very first segment I made on TV in 1994 entailed a visit to a trailer in western Montana in which two men in Nazi-style outfits explained God's cosmic plan for different races to be banished to separate planets. Nearly thirty years later, I'm ploughing the same furrow, though thanks to the web and the rise of nativism, you don't have to travel nearly so far to hear similar views. More customer-friendly versions are being peddled on laptops and phones in bedrooms around the world and there is a generation of young people for whom the idea of embracing edgy far-right content and tongue-in-cheek and not-so-tongue-in-cheek racism carries a countercultural cachet as a break from the brainwashed boredom of Normie-dom.

Nick Fuentes is the avatar of this movement. He was at Charlottesville, Virginia, at the Unite the Right rally, arriving the day after a parade of white racists marched with tiki torches and chanted 'You will not replace us' and 'Jews will not replace us' and where the anti-racist demonstrator Heather Heyer lost her life after a deranged white nationalist drove his car into a crowd. In the wake of Charlottesville, with the movement discredited in the eyes of anyone remotely mainstream, Fuentes rebranded himself an 'America First' nationalist. He discouraged followers from using imagery that was too explicitly Nazi-tinged, impressing on them the need to be 'optical', while on a nightly streaming show he continued to express coded – and not so coded – white-nationalist ideas about there being a problem with Jewish power and black crime. Gradually, he cultivated a large following of maladapted teenagers and twenty-somethings who call themselves 'Groypers' and who loved Nick for his cheeky persona, modelled on popular YouTubers, as much as for his politics.

And so to Orlando, to commence filming on what we are calling the 'dissident right' project, also known as 'radicals', which, like the Florida rap one, we had been forced to put on ice nearly a year ago by the sudden onset of a global pandemic. It was a short shoot, only three days, and the occasion for it was a conference Nick was hosting at a hotel. The event – called AFPAC, for America First Political Action Committee – was happening at the same time and in the same city as CPAC, which is the big Republican conference. Trump is attending that one. It was a bit like the Edinburgh Festival and the Fringe. Except, in the case of AFPAC, it was the extremist fringe.

The night before I left, Nancy and I watched a horror film called *Sinister*, with Arthur, *not* with Ray – we're pretty lax though I'd like to think not actively sociopathic. It's about a struggling writer who finds a box of old tapes, which prefigure the daughter becoming – spoiler alert – possessed by an ancient Babylonian deity called Bughuul and killing the rest of the family. It may say something about Covid times that the scenario did not seem that far removed from reality.

The following morning, knowing I had to leave, I came down with Ray, and denying him his iPad heard in return his new catchphrase: 'Aagh! You're the worst!' Nancy emerged a bit later.

'Good morning, angry lady,' I said.

'I *am* angry. Fifteen years of this, Louis.'

'I don't want it to go on like this any more than you do. I'm making a commitment. I want to be around more.'

'I'll believe it when I see it.'

From the airport, I wrote to Art: **By the power of B'ghoul, eater**

of children, I command you to be good for Mum. He replied: **It's spelled Bughuul.**

After the eight-hour flight – arriving in Miami in the evening – I had a four-hour car ride to the hotel in Orlando. In the back of the car, as I was being driven, I caught up on some reading on Fuentes and America First. Then the phone pinged. Messages coming in from Nancy saying she and Ray were awake. It was three in the morning in London but Ray had worms and they were preventing him from sleeping. I commiserated, then tried to help by googling chemists in NW6 to find somewhere they could get the medicine, Ovex, noticing for the first time in my life that there seem to be no twenty-four-hour chemists anywhere in London. Then I tried Amazon and other mail-order options. Nothing doing. I felt like ground control trying to repair a leak on the space station – Nancy and Ray slowly running out of oxygen. Eventually, she rang off and close to midnight I arrived at my hotel.

The event turned out to be a gathering of the tribes, for pale young men in suits, college Republican types, a handful of full-bore misfits dressed up in outfits from another era, like barbershop quartet singers in straw boaters with oiled moustaches, about five women, three black people, and a smattering of alt-right celebrities. The term of art for many of the attendees would be 'incel', the portmanteau derived from 'involuntary celibate', the self-designation used by denizens of the darker parts of the Internet who are unable to find female companionship.

Fuentes presided over his group, godlike amid the beta hordes, skinny but handsome, like an undernourished gamer-nerd JFK tribute act, with a Cheshire Cat grin so broad that it narrows his eyes. I'd bumped into him crossing the lobby of his hotel. He was wearing a Hawaiian shirt and shorts, in holiday mode, accompanied by a young, college-age friend called Jaden. Jaden was a fellow Groyper. He'd been kicked out of college, I'd been told, for sending a tweet in the wake of the BLM movement, saying, 'Congratulations to George Floyd on one month drug free.' I fell into step with them, then spent the afternoon in Fuentes's retinue as he inspected the preparations for the event in the Hilton banqueting hall: pale young guys in masks were setting up, laying tables, putting out promotional stickers of the Groyper logo – a fat cartoon frog. Their faces were hard to read, they were mainly wearing masks, but they had the air of conservative gamer boys in T-shirts.

I interviewed as we went. Fuentes enjoys debate and the challenge for me was to hold off getting too deep in the conversation. I was there to follow the action and not disappear into the weeds for a discussion of his views on US foreign policy and big tech deplatforming – there would be plenty of time on future shoot days to push harder on his track record of extreme statements and his real beliefs. In fact, he is adept at positioning himself as vaguely mainstream, an old-fashioned conservative who tells it like it is. Over everything was the looming shadow of 6 January and the attack on the Capitol. The FBI was investigating him, he said. He'd been there but had stayed outside – the man in the congressional office behind Baked Alaska, depicted in a widely shared photo, who looked like Nick, was someone else. The media had overhyped the whole occasion, he said. It was a simple protest, not that many people had got inside, and anyway, why shouldn't they be there, it was 'the people's house'.

This was all delivered with a little twinkle of deniability.

We had lunch together, off camera, in an open-air mall in the shadow of a huge Ferris wheel, passing the time with conversation about food and Chicago, where he was born and raised, and other people in 'the movement'. Loud music was playing and every fifteen minutes or so a colourful toy train carrying kids would pass by.

'We should film you on that,' I said. 'Good optics.'

'*Bad* optics,' he said.

Late in the day, just before we called it a night, one or two of Nick's more fringe beliefs peeped out. He'd prefer if women didn't have the right to vote, he said. Civilization had started its decline with female suffrage. Women in general couldn't be in the inner circle of the movement. This was followed by a random reference to the evil bigwigs who were, as he saw it, screwing up society. 'They're not *all* Jews,' he said, again with an air of naughty humour.

Then the following day – the main event. In the morning, Nick was hard to summon on the phone so we slunk into the venue having arranged an interview with one of his satellites, a Hispanic filmmaker named Stephen Martinez, then loitered in the vicinity picking off interviews with other attendees. Through the afternoon, the venue filled up, many of them dweeby guys, none too keen to speak to – or even be filmed by – a member of the liberal lamestream media, but there was an undoubted May Ball energy to the occasion. Fuentes emerged late afternoon, his time taken up posing for photos with fans who had paid for the privilege, in a manner a little reminiscent of Pooh Sheisty on his bus at the car show or indeed L. Theroux on his Australian tour. I stalked about trying to find consenting interviewees. A handful of people in the audience – three or four – recognized me. 'Oh yeah, I've seen your documentaries. *Wacky Weekends?*' One, referring at random to an old programme I'd made about trophy hunting in Africa, said without preamble, 'Why didn't you shoot the warthog?'

When the time came for speeches, the auditorium darkened. Slick introductory packages had been prepared. Fuentes, the headliner, was preceded by a stylish hype video showing him speaking through a bullhorn at rallies and Stop the Steal events. There were fast cuts and loud music – the look they were going for was latter-day Che Guevara, shot from below, striking street-fighter barricade-storming poses. Then he took to the stage to wild applause, launching into his variation on themes Trump popularized in 2016 – closing borders and decrying globalists and Washington elites – combined with moments of edgelord provocation. Fuentes has made his career out of out-flanking Republicans from the right, and he spent much of his time making fun of right-wingers for not being right-wing enough. But what was maybe most striking was his poise, his relaxed insouciant air, and his command of the crowd, his ability to activate them with red-meat moments. 'White people are tired of being bullied,' he said at one point. Chants of 'America First' and 'Christ is King' went through the audience like electricity. In the background was a feeling that this was the insurgent army of a radical Trump base. A coalition of religious zealots, incels, gamers, conspiracy theorists and lost boys.

What was also in my head was the sense of being back in the saddle. A campaign that had been planned more than a year earlier, and that was a distant lineal descendant of an idea I'd worked on in 2017, about the far-right Internet edgelords who claimed to have memed Trump into the presidency, was now in effect more than four years later. I was back in the fray.

I was conscious, too, of how old I was – a fifty-year-old amid the gamer boys. There was a time when I'd been the young one and the stories had been populated by the middle-aged. Now it was the reverse. And the world had changed so much. Not just from Covid, but from the other viruses: populism, nativism, misogyny, and by their antibodies: progressivism, wokeness, sensitivity. And where did I stand? A white person telling a story about white tribal identity? And what was my responsibility, giving airtime to people who were something between Froot Loops and legit, as they pirouetted on the edge of white nationalism, no longer in trailers in Montana but in homes near you and in palaces of government? I imagined a backlash to the film, whenever it came out. I might have to stay off Twitter for a bit. Weather the storm. No point playing it safe, dodging controversy. And, then catastrophizing in typical style, I thought: *If it's the end it's the end.*

On the last day, with scant minutes to spare, we shot a sequence of Nick driving up in a convertible sports car, parking outside the hotel where they are hosting CPAC – the more mainstream though in fact still very right-wing political convention from which Nick's been banned for extremism – and stepping out like an incel Alain Delon. His stereo was playing Jay-Z at loud volume – his love of rap, and Kanye especially, is one of Nick's more confusing and disruptive bits of political signalling. A rapture bordering on ecstasy was legible on the faces of the twenty or so America Firsters who were there to greet him and they proceeded to stage a slightly limp guerrilla protest, 'attempting' (not very hard) to enter the CPAC conference, stomping on a surgical mask, being turned away, and driving off.

And that was that. I was due at the airport and there followed an overnight flight back to Heathrow, and an interminable near-stationary queue at immigration that took an hour or more to move through. I passed the time on a long call about our Joe Exotic project and fixes and how we structure it. We have been in a phase of thinking it should be two hour-long programmes, given that we have a complicated mix of material – the archive from my visit in 2011, the new stuff we shot, news footage to explain what happened in the interim with his murder-for-hire case, then the strange twist of having the *Tiger King* production team trying to spike our guns. It's a lot to deal with, but now it seems likely it will work better as a single ninety-minute film, which is also what the channel appears to want, so having lobbied hard in one direction I am now in the position of reversing course.

Midway through discussing this, still stuck in the queue, my battery died.

Taxi back to north-west London. Kissed and hugged Nancy,

thanked her for holding the fort, and made tea for both of us. When Ray arrived back from school, we played Roblox together – an online platform with user-generated games where the avatars are weird blockmen like the Honeywell advert from the eighties. The user names all sound like SoundCloud rap names: Trecherous999 is Ray's, his friend's is DarkAngel5000.

In other news, Marce texted to say he's had the Oxford jab. **Thank you, NHS**, he wrote on the family WhatsApp. Where is my jab? He is only two years older than me. Does my status as the Dame Vera Lynn of Lockdown Podcasting™ mean nothing?

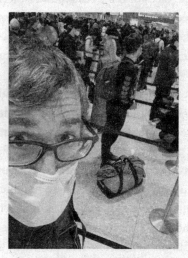

Welcome home!

Tuesday 2 March

A birthday card arrived for Arthur from my dad. Art's birthday was two weeks ago, but better late than never. The card contained fifty euros.

I asked Nancy, 'Why do you suppose he sent euros?'

'I guess he didn't have any pounds.'

'I only got forty euros,' Jack said.

I offered to change the money

'It's forty-three pounds. I checked,' Art said.

Then Jack said, 'Do you know which currency is worth most? The Koo-whitey money.'

'Wait, what?'

'The Kuwaiti dinar?' Nancy said.

'Yes. Why are you laughing? It's literally the richest currency you can get, unlike the pound, which is the most noob currency.'

Ray seemed tired after his school day. He played Imaginext for a while, then vegged in front of the TV. After the big guys had had supper, Jack went in and I heard Ray's voice shout, 'Go fucking away!'

A Ray first.

Monday 8 March

Officially, the kids are back at school today. Big moment. The weather's cold and our energy monitor continuing to cause anxiety because it looks like we are haemorrhaging gas and electricity at a crazy rate. Ten, twelve pounds per day. Can this be right? Surely it's broken? I turn lights off, install low-energy bulbs, acquire a German-engineered remote access system. Yet I wake up at 7.30 and we're already two pounds down. Is it possible the monitor itself is consuming vast quantities of energy?

Jack's not yet back at school, as it's a staggered start, but I took Ray in – he'd been on the iPad since about 7.30 while I was washing-up. He cycled at breakneck speed and then ran in with no fuss, excited to be part of a well-attended school again.

Spent the day on Zoom calls working on Joe Exotic, trying to sort out the first half. For several hours I pushed it into a structure that felt like it was on the verge of working if we could just torture the dialogue into saying what it needed to, until late in the day we watched the cut back and it was *still* not working and I was thinking, *I'm out of ideas, I've fucked this up, I've led the team down a cul-de-sac and now I don't know what to do*, and I gave in, and accepted my plan had been wrong. We reverted to an earlier version that works a million times better.

There's a viewing on Friday with a channel executive that can't be moved.

Ray arrived home around six, dropped off by his childminder, and skipped inside and threw his satchel at the sofa.

'How was it being back at school with all the other children, Ray?'

'Good.'

'Was it good or are you just saying that?'

'Fantastic,' he said, with an air of decision.

Tuesday 9 March

Spring is here. From my window I can see the hawthorn and the apple blossom. Today was Jack's first day back. In his uniform like a straitjacket, he went off without a fuss. Ray's drop-off was more crowded today. A ragged queue outside the school, Ray on his bike jockeying past pedestrians on the pavement. He ran in again, no clinging, and I cycled back for a long session with the Joe Exotic edit via Zoom.

When Jack arrived home after school, I asked how it had felt.

'Good. Kind of weird but kind of normal.'

Wednesday 10 March

Calls, Zooms, viewings of cuts. Do you care? At 1 hour 48 minutes the Joe Exotic film is showing signs of working. We have three editors on it. It starts with a bang now and there is a logic to the flow of material and we've been able to work in more of the 2011 footage, which is the star of the show, containing as it does so much candid material with Joe . . . Pre-title with Trump press conference, then me at home, letter from Joe, recap, title, Joe's lawyers 2020, 2011 material about park, Carole and Howard . . . And the new bits Emma the editor has worked in of Joe in lighter mode – playing with animals, joking, talking about staff – all give the film a sense of space and play. It slightly falls off a cliff in the second half when *Tiger King* enters the picture. Maybe that is in the nature of the material. The thread slackens – we need to tighten and add urgency. Losing eighteen minutes should help.

Will life ever be sane again? Life is somewhat sane. And somewhat not. The government health guru Chris Whitty said there would be another surge in the late summer if all restrictions are lifted on 21 June as has been mentioned. But no lockdown planned? I don't know. I can't keep up. He said: 'Even when people are fully vaccinated, a significant minority, it's not large but a significant minority, do go on to get significant disease. It's not zero.'

We are alive, even though I barely leave the house except to get milk and wine and dishwasher tablets. I don't watch TV. I work and play with the kids and cook and do laundry and watch cuts and drink and work. But some people are going into work. Nancy says she's going in tomorrow.

Spring may be here but it doesn't feel like it. Rain and wind are shaking the eucalyptus.

Thursday 11 March

Nancy went into the office. I was at home on my own for the first time in many days, sitting on Zooms, making more cuts and fixes to the Joe film.

I made a sausage and red pepper pasta thing based on an adaptation of a recipe I found by googling the random selection of ingredients that were in the fridge. After supper I walked down to the Co-op with Jack, me mainly in silence, brooding, thinking about the Joe Exotic cut and what I could have done differently. I wondered whether we should have filmed a trip his campaign team made to Washington DC in January to advocate for a pardon from Trump. His lawyer, Francisco, had asked us along. Why hadn't we gone? It might have been funny – we'd have crossed paths with the *Tiger King* crew and it could have been like a real-life version of the news team gang fight in *Anchorman*. The trip had been on the same day as the Capitol riots, which means instead of filming I was getting drunk and watching a frozen frog defrost on TV. The decision had been taken, in any case – there was no going back, so I should probably try to stop thinking about it. But still, it was hard to ignore and in hindsight it was so obvious that was the scene that might have taken us over the edge. The one people talked about.

Friday 12 March

High-tempo race to ready the Joe Exotic cut for a 4 p.m. remote viewing for the BBC commissioner. A cut came in in the middle of last night. A Zoom meeting at 8.15 in the morning to discuss last-minute nips and tucks, which I didn't make due to drop-off. I joined at 9 a.m. and then recorded some last-minute voice-over lines.

'It's really good,' said the commissioner, when the call finally happened. Her only major notes are to do with how we handle the material around the *Tiger King* series. A scene in which Joe's niece Chealsi, protective of the dignity of her Oklahoma compatriots and imputing metropolitan disdain to the *Tiger King* directors, claims, possibly erroneously, 'They got one guy drunk . . . They filmed [Joe's husband] John Finlay with his shirt off. Who does that?'

'I just can't help thinking, haven't we all filmed someone with their shirt off?' the commissioner said.

'Well, to be fair, they asked John Finlay to take his shirt off,' Jack said. 'Or at least that's what John Finlay has said. But I know what you mean.'

'I filmed a neo-Nazi who was drunk,' I allowed. 'I definitely didn't *get him drunk*, but I bought the alcohol and I was thinking, *It'll be great if he gets drunk.*'

Everyone is, I think, conscious of bad or dodgy choices we might have made in the past; disgruntled former subjects, non-textbook decisions, small payments and editorial missteps, but also there is a laudable wish not to be pious.

After the call, I said to our team, 'I'm not trying to be the documentary ethics purist. It's easy to be holier than thou. I'm more in the seventies cop way of thinking, the guy who breaks rules and gets results. If you did everything completely by the book, honest to god, no good films would get made.'

Honest to god, I don't know if I meant this as I said it.

Saturday 13 March

Late in the evening, in bed, I was seized by a sudden curiosity. On my phone, I googled, 'Coterie Cafe', the beleaguered little place with the sad-faced manager in our old Shepherd's Bush office building. I found an Instagram account. 'Contemporary cafe & bar serving up healthy, inventive gourmet food, drinks & cocktails,' it said. The account looked well tended. The photos were beautiful and recently added: 'Jackfruit tacos'. 'Tropical passionfruit popsicles'. 'Lemon and mascarpone tart'. They're doing fine.

Sunday 14 March

Yesterday, on the news, a judge awarded $27 million to the family of George Floyd. The largest pre-trial payout to a family in US history. The criminal trial of Derek Chauvin, the cop who killed him, still to take place. On WhatsApp, a message from Arron: **BTW it's the one-year anniversary of [our BBC commissioner] calling and saying 'I don't think you can get on the plane' for the first time.**

Nancy has had a text saying she can get the jab. She qualifies due to having asthma. One of her brothers, who is a carer, is already vaccinated. Marce's wife too. Fifty-two Covid deaths today. Back in late January there were over 1,000 a day.

Monday 15 March

Ray drop-off. Wicks. Calls. Lunch. Calls. Emails. Every day that the kids are at school feels like a privilege. You sit at your desk and look out of the window and breathe and listen to the quiet.

Across the water in Italy and France there are corona surges that are weirdly reminiscent of last year. New restrictions are coming into force. The vaccines haven't arrived in sufficient quantities, an Italian virologist said. At the same time, numerous countries are pausing the AstraZeneca roll-out over fears it causes blood clots.

I just looked up the total number of global deaths. It is 2.66 million. Order of ranking of countries for deaths in absolute numbers, with worst first, is: USA, Brazil, India, Russia, the UK.

Tuesday 16 March

In the morning, on the radio, an item about a year with corona. They interviewed a historian who said the twenty-first century would be written as 'BC' and 'AC'. Before and after Covid-19. Did he still believe this? the woman asked. Yes, he said. The world was very different now. Exactly how was hard to discern, because at the point the historian was about to explain Nancy came in and turned the radio down because she was looking for her phone and was ringing it, but I suppose he was going to acknowledge the massive loss of life and the steep downturns in the economies and the renewed awareness of the precariousness of our position on Earth. Or maybe not. Maybe he was going to say something else. *We may never know.*

Mid-morning, on a conference call about Joe Exotic and phrasing and rewrites and trims, I got a text saying I could make an NHS vaccination appointment. I followed the link and within a minute of finger work on my phone I was booked in for Saturday at 12.15. For a begrudging moment, given how much they got wrong, I thanked the government for getting it right on this, and also the NHS and whoever else it is that made the vaccinations available in large quantities, meaning largely healthy, slightly bourbon-ravaged fifty-year-old me is getting jabbed while many other countries are panicked and running short. In Israel, they are opening up concerts and public events to people who have vaccination passports. They say this is what the future may look like.

The Internet went down the rest of the day, problems on the road or the pipes – the neighbours were complaining they too had lost signal. I had to use a weak to non-existent 3G, one or two bars, a tiny piddling trickle of data. I felt like I'd been miniaturized, a six-inch-high man with a piping voice having to join Zoom calls via a regular audio call to someone's phone and being put on speaker, feeding in notes, not knowing how much I was being heard. *The scene with the bear is still playing a bit long.* No TV, no radio, no smart speaker, everything's connected to the Internet. I couldn't even turn the heating down. Well, I could. I just couldn't do it from my phone.

The channel has said they don't like 'I Shot Joe Exotic' as the title. A title I love. It suggests I'm claiming ownership of the story, they say. I *am* claiming ownership of the story, I wanted to say. They said, What about 'Joe Exotic and Me'? I want to reply: What about 'A Film About A Man'? If we want to be super-lame, let's go all in.

Wednesday 17 March

I was interviewed by Troy Deeney in the morning for a new podcast he's doing. I hosted him on *Grounded* back in May of last year, plus he'd helped me by forwarding on a message to Anthony Joshua in November, when I was trying to get him on my podcast, so I owed him a favour. One hand washes the other. At eleven, I got on calls with the Joe Exotic editor and looked at comm lines and trims. The announcement of the programme went out early this morning in a press release of calculated blandness that said almost nothing about what is in it, the idea being not to kick up too much pre-emptive fuss from the *Tiger King* lawyers. The story has been picked up in the *Hollywood Reporter*, *Deadline*, all the tabloids.

Nancy made a sausage carbonara dish while I looked at emails at my computer. One had come in from a woman who said she runs Joe Exotic's social media account and he wanted to be in touch. I drafted an email in response saying I wasn't allowed to make contact with Joe, due to the legal agreement he signed with the *Tiger King* team. Then I realized I might be legally prohibited from sending it and checked with Arron to see if he could check with the lawyers. Answer: better not to send.

A new cut came in, with final tweaks and voice-over changes and trims. After supper I walked down to the Co-op with Jack, who was intent on getting some frozen mango for a smoothie he had planned. For a while we went in silence. I was preoccupied, thinking about work. Jack asked about mockumentaries. What were they? I tried to explain. A film and TV genre that mimics the grammar of documentaries. But they're fake. 'It's hard to get right,' I said, 'because the entire point of documentaries is that you forgive the limitations of what you see – the fact that it's muted or off-camera or not very well shot – because of the knowledge that it's real and you focus on enjoying the subtleties of texture. There are very few good mockumentaries. *Spinal Tap* may be the only one.'

There were the usual homeless men outside the Sainsbury's and the Co-op.

'All right, LT?' said the man called Khan, outside the Co-op. 'Can you help me out?'

'I could buy you some food or drink if you like?'

'I need money for a B and B,' he said.

'I'll catch you on the way out.'

We bought our items – fruit, veg, booze. Frozen mangos they turned out not to have.

Coming out, having made a decision, I gave Khan ten pounds. 'This covers me for the next few visits,' I said.

Back at the house, with the light lowering behind the eucalyptus, the kids played out back, Jack, for once, not teasing Ray, but pushing him back and forth on a skateboard, while Arthur bounced on a trampoline at the end of the garden.

'Well, this makes a change,' I said to Nancy. 'A temporary truce between the trenches.'

'Don't jinx it,' she said.

A little later, I took Ray upstairs where we read a Trolls-themed book, with objects hidden in the pictures: Can you find the nine mushrooms? The ten doughnuts? The twenty candy canes? Nancy called in from outside the door, 'You should have lights *off* now. It's nearly nine.' We still had some way to go, and I pretended to find the objects to speed it along. 'Oh, look, there's the cane! In the tree!'

'Where?'

'Never mind! Next page!'

I kissed him goodnight. 'You're a lifesaver,' he said. A phrase he picked up somewhere. I don't think he knows what it means.

This is my last entry. I'm sitting here almost a year to the day I started, with a glass of wine next to me. Life goes on. There are outbreaks and there are shortages and there are signs of hope. We are nearly three million fewer through corona, with the end still not in sight, and secondary pandemics rippling out in unseen ways, crises of poverty and the mental health of those who struggled in lockdown – anxiety, depression, eating disorders. We have an idea of what the future may look like. Different and the same, better and worse, and for now I'm going to let it be and sip my wine and count myself grateful for every day that comes.

Epilogue

Going Viral

A little before midday, on a Saturday in late March, I cycled down to Willesden Health Centre on Robson Road, having stopped off at the local corner shop to buy a mask because I'd forgotten to bring one, chained up my bike and went inside to be greeted by a woman in a high-vis jacket standing in the lobby. 'Here for the vaccination?' she said.

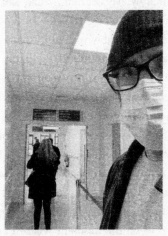

Getting vaxxed.

From there it was a chain of cheery volunteers, 'if you wouldn't mind moving down to my colleague down there?', gelling of hands, checking of papers laid out on folding tables – someone at one point gave me a raffle ticket – until, a few minutes after arriving, I was inside a large clinical room, where a middle-aged Irish nurse who had just come on duty explained it would be 'the Oxford'.

'You'll be scheduled for the second one between six and twelve weeks. But there are some issues with supply as you probably know.' She held out a little card. 'This is not the passport but it does say you've had the jab and what batch you've had so you'll want to hold on to it. They're still engineering the vaccine to keep it up to date, so it may be that there'll be another we all have to have in the autumn.'

'Little prick,' she said. 'There you go. Now you're as brave as Boris Johnson.'

I had a weird few weeks after the vaccination. One night, in April, I woke up in the small hours feeling out of sorts and uncharacteristically melancholy. My ordinary small worries loomed large in the quiet of the night. I thought about my alcohol consumption and the havoc it was presumably wreaking on my body, about dying early, my life drifting away, not getting to see my children grow up due to liver failure or other booze-related health issues, my organs shrivelling or maybe swelling, cracking, flaking, growing spongey, the exact medical details were unclear. Personal failures crowded my head like ghosts. Wasn't I basically a pretty lousy person? Not a very considerate friend? Didn't call my dad often. Not very thoughtful to my mum. An impatient and work-preoccupied father. What in fact did I contribute to the world, other than making documentaries, which was a basically narcissistic endeavour?

This is supposed to be the moment where I say I dedicated my life to Christ that night and never looked back. I didn't do that. But over the following few days I eased up on the boozing, feeling some combination of virtuous and bored, turning in at 10 p.m. after three cups of herbal tea. I also called and had a nice chat with my dad.

On Easter Monday, *Shooting Joe Exotic* went out on BBC Two, creating a small ripple of appreciation among the million or so who watched; Twitter not exactly in meltdown – no memes in evidence, no celebrities dressing up in mullet wigs, just a couple of texts from my mum and my brother.

Reviews were mainly positive, several one might describe as *glowing*, one or two one might describe as *grudging* – two stars in the *Telegraph*, and the phrase 'sour grapes' was used in connection with my take on *Tiger King*. Thereafter, the wording of the article made visits to my brainspace like a comet with a three-day orbit, and I inadvertently memorized the name of the reviewer. As the weeks went by, work continued on my other projects – I made follow-up trips for dissident right and Florida rap and planned towards filming a third documentary about #MeToo coming to porn. The series that had come to be known as *Gods of Snooker* came to air to great reviews – the *New Statesman* called it a masterpiece. The Jeremy Bamber series, mostly filmed now, took shape in the edit, the Joe Wicks documentary Spider-Man-lunged towards its first shoot days, and other Mindhouse singles and series prepared to launch, or sputtered out, or were held back while technical difficulties were figured out.

And so here we are, halfway through the epilogue, at the end of the book, at that point when you can feel a slackening of the pace. The main action has concluded, the characters are on stage but out of breath after the finale, their hands raised to the rafters, and we can be confident there will be no further musical numbers. Only life, being life, isn't always like that. In late May, a few days after my birthday, possibly via Ray and a trip to the park and an ice cream or through some other pathway, a string of Covid infections took place. Family members, friends and loved ones tumbled in a trail like dominoes: Arthur, Jack, my mum, her other half Michael, my nephew and niece, two of Arthur's friends and possibly assorted other people I don't even know all seemed to fall victim to the latest iteration of the virus, the 'Delta variant', also dubbed 'the Indian variant', imported to these shores partly owing – it was said – to a two-week delay on locking-down borders, possibly because – it was alleged – Boris Johnson had an upcoming trade trip to India.

More infectious, more likely to be passed on by children – for our kids, their tango with the Delta involved a headache, a sore throat, some vomiting and listlessness. The symptoms didn't last long – a couple of days. A friend of Arthur's suffered significantly more: bedridden for nearly a week, with chest pains. For my mum and Michael, their doses of the vaccine appeared to do the trick; they mentioned mild ailments that they said were not vastly different from the ordinary afflictions of old age. Michael complained of a dry mouth and loss of taste. My mum had her doubts about whether Michael really had the virus, given by now there had been five or six false alarms, and even after it was confirmed using a test acquired at Boots, she continued to suspect he might be malingering.

Mirabile dictu, the Dame Vera Lynn of Lockdown Podcasting™ was by this point double-vaxxed – his national morale-lifting gifts mercifully unscathed by any discernible Covid symptoms, other than possibly a day or two of grumpiness, indistinguishable from his normal personality.

But for the singly vaxxed Mrs LT – whose second jab was only days away when she was taken down – the Covid assault came on more vengefully, starting with shivery coldness, a sore throat, strange wind, produced mainly by mouth, and a growing breathlessness, culminating one awful sleepless Saturday night in her waking me in a panic because she found she was incapable of deep breaths, which was in turn creating a feedback loop of anxiety and panic.

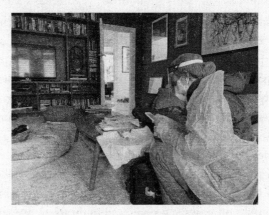

A Covid tester calls.

Asthma runs in Nancy's family – her grandmother died from an attack before Nancy was born, when she would have been around Nancy's age now – and all this, though unspoken, was in the background to our concern that night. 'I'm really frightened,' she said, and we held each other. I tried to offer advice, remembering that her brother had mentioned that when he'd struggled to breathe for two nights he'd stayed very still. I told her she looked OK – which she did: there was colour in her face. She said that helped to calm her. I tried to take her mind elsewhere, discouraging her from reading up on symptoms. It was all a little reminiscent of when our first child was born, and holding her hand through the labour. We went downstairs and I made camomile tea. We got through the night.

The following morning, she was feeling nauseous. She vomited. Her breathing was still shallow and she called an NHS helpline. An ambulance came, and she walked out and climbed inside as Ray watched, too little to know what it portended, but undoubtedly noticing something out of the ordinary. Around midday I picked her up from the hospital – she'd had some tests and the staff were satisfied she was getting enough air. Over the following week, she continued to struggle, enfeebled and breathless, incapable of anything requiring exertion, but the worst of it was a feeling of bleakness, which I had to remind her was a symptom of the condition, and not a reflection of our real life. The second week was marginally worse. She was still unable to go into work, lacking breath, demoralized, and finding it hard to switch off at home, preoccupied with her commitments to our company. Then gradually she mended. Day by day she felt a little better,

And what about you? How are you feeling? Are you in lockdown now? Are you back to normal, with only vestigial measures remaining, like masks on buses and tubes and in theatres? Are you far in the future wearing an Elon Musk brain chip, living in a sim run by Chinese oligarchs, and is the virus a distant memory? As I write this it is 19 July 2021. The government has removed all the restrictions that were in place in England – including mask-wearing and social distancing – and decided to dub the event 'Freedom Day', in an act of hubris reminiscent of George W. Bush in 2003, when he landed on an aircraft carrier and declared, apropos of the US invasion of Iraq, 'Mission Accomplished', presaging an orgy of bloodletting and destruction that has never completely abated. The virus is once again surging. Hospitalizations are spiking, though the death rate for now remains flat. The word of the week is 'ping' – as in, being 'pinged' by the government Track and Trace app and told to self-isolate. So many people are being pinged, huge holes have appeared in the workforce, and there is a general feeling that the pinging is so metastatic as to be unsustainable. There are reports of mass non-compliance with the pinging and rampant erasing of the app. Still, the feeling abroad, when I stick my wet finger in the wind, is that for the UK at least the very worst may be behind us. There is a wary sense that we are getting back towards some kind of normal, coming back to life like a patient awaking from a coma, learning to walk again, though unsure what exactly lies at the end of the road, whether we will ever dance our funky robot moves the way we used to or stand a realistic chance of winning *Strictly*.

'We all have strength enough to endure the misfortunes of others.' So said the French aphorist and arch-cynic La Rochefoucauld.

A world remade by catastrophe and death has reminded us of the human power to handle tragedy, especially other people's. Like a crowded restaurant filling with smoke, what has been striking in Covid World isn't the pulling together or the malice, the untapped reserves of resilience or nastiness, it is the sense of hysteria, the noise, the confusion – shouts of anger and fear and a contagious feeling of panic as everyone rushes in different directions looking for the door. One would hope that the levelling effect of a disease notionally catchable by anyone would create a democratic feeling of shared struggle. *We're all in this together* was the early catchphrase. But this turned out not always to be true: the poor suffered more, the crowded-in-houses suffered more, the parents who worked and couldn't keep up and worried about money with young kids out of school suffered more. For a reality-show president, his case of Covid arrived with the most complete battery of medical support available to humankind. So too for a rumple-haired Old Etonian. Others, the less lucky ones, languished alone and died. But, let it be said, the spiralling death toll and Trump's fact-blind unwilling-ness to take measures to stop the spread did have the side effect of losing him his job. The man addicted to calling out 'fake news' found there was a limit to his ability to use tweets to arrange reality to his needs. A coronavirus called by any other name aerosolizes just as effectively.

'Strange times' was another phrase. The idea that this was an aberration, a moment of singular weirdness. But I tend to think the real lesson may be the opposite: Covid wasn't a lightning strike of misfortune, it was a bill coming due. The latest and maybe not even the most menacing of a number of assailants, global in scale, invading our homes, making our lives worse, all of them, in different ways, of our own making. The miracle of the modern world, our domination of the planet, has a price. An instantaneous communication system that allows *stuff* – data, products, organic matter – to travel the world at lightning speed and which we've deployed to fulfil our every passing need, has bitten us back, forcing us to reckon with our own actions as we feed a set of inborn appetites every bit as primitive as they were 30,000 years ago: food, sex, entertainment, ego. And so we find ourselves attacked by monsters that are more or less of our creation: tribal insanity, disinformation, metastatic viruses, global warming, data-harvesting apps that weaponize our urge to be distracted, albums by Ed Sheeran. Just joking. I quite like Ed Sheeran.

I should mention, by the way, that investigations are ongoing as to whether the Covid pandemic *was* the result of someone chowing down on a pangolin burger – as was initially thought – or whether it was in fact due to a lab leak at the Wuhan Institute of Virology. This theory – that a worker at the specialist viral lab that just happens to be situated at the source of the pandemic unintentionally released the virus – had been mooted early in 2020 and written off by mainstream media as a conspiracy theory and banned from Facebook, reminding us that the label 'fake news' is sometimes in the eye of the beholder, and that yet another of our adversaries is the overly complacent policing of supposedly heretical views.

In the midst of the various global monsters, we make the best choices we can. For me, the assault of the virus meant a reset in the most local sense: a grand adventure at home, a stationary version of those life-changing round-the-world trips families sometimes take. Instead of investigating Kathmandu or South America, we were travelling from room to room in our socks, trying not to step on Lego bricks.

I lived life at a different pace. I started a company. It did well. I was around more for my kids, which made me realize I wanted to be away less. I got to know my wife in a different way, no longer simply loving her and fancying her but also admiring her as a collaborator and a creative partner.

Many times during the various lockdowns, in the madness and stress occasioned by being cooped-up, I wondered if I might be a terrible dad. It's not the first time I've had the thought. But I'd like to think that those conscience-pricks are the evidence of caring and wanting to do better. And what I do know is that the relentlessness of trying to be an OK parent is far harder than any programme I've made. I've got three Baftas. I'm not mentioning it gratuitously. OK. I am. Bafta, Bafta, Bafta. Three of them. The point is, if there were awards for being a parent, I'm not saying I would win one – I definitely wouldn't – but the amount of work it would *take* to win one puts my Baftas in the shithouse, with apologies to the Academy. Why am I even telling you this? For all I know you have six children who you homeschool, and they all speak fluent Latin and knit their own yogurt and don't even know what YouTube *is*. But from where I'm sitting, holy shit, it is hard. It is *so* hard. And that is in the best of times, and these were not the best of times.

The desire to bear witness to the angst of normal family life is part of why I started writing this book. I look back and I'm embarrassed at how much of what is on display in these pages is pain and arguing and me being a dick. But I'd also like to think that what really underlies all that stress and bickering is love. They say, about life, that it's what happens when you're busy making other plans. Well, I wonder if, with love, it may be something similar: that it's all the things we think it is *not*. It doesn't land on us from somewhere. It isn't separate. It exists in everything we do, choices we make, investments of time and energy. Maybe instead of an emotion it is better to think of love as something we practise. In fact, at the risk of really disappearing into the realm of Hallmark cards,

I'd say the heart is a muscle. Something you can exercise and grow. And when I consider the pain of everything we've been through and how much we all took on and are still taking on, that's what I'd like to dwell on: that the pain was the exertion of our hearts as they worked and grew stronger.

All through the three lockdowns, the metaphor that came to mind was of a desert island. I'd been marooned with my family in the middle of an indifferent sea, in a vast Bear Grylls-style bivouac, only with four bedrooms, and equipped with TV and electricity and hot and cold running water and limitless supplies of food and booze and video games.

Now we are on a rescue vessel, and the island is growing small on the horizon, and I wave goodbye to the place that was our home for all those months, and I feel a little sorry to go – a part of me doesn't want to face the world again, knowing how much of myself I'm leaving behind, and there is also a wary recognition that it's possible we may be going back – but the greatest part sees something deeper, that we are stronger for what we have been through, whatever happens next.

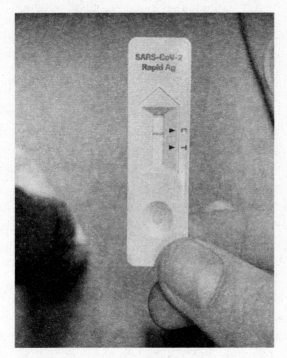

Negative.

Read on for the prologue from Louis Theroux's
acclaimed autobiography

Gotta Get Theroux This

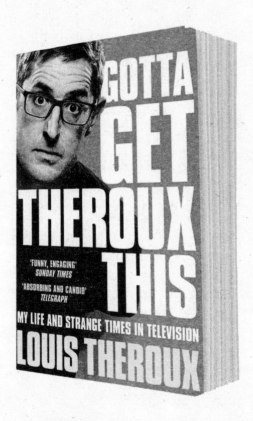

Prologue

Sensual Eating

Though I knew him to be a business executive and samba instructor, the poised man who came to the door in his t-shirt and pyjama bottoms, with his well-tended white beard and faint air of naughtiness, looked more like the sensei at an erotic dojo.

I was a little out of breath. The house – tall, with wooden decks around it – stood on the side of a pine-covered slope on a street on the edge of Portland, Oregon, and I'd had to climb a steep drive in inappropriate leather footwear to get there, being met at the top by Cliff, my host.

He ushered me inside – my crew followed behind – and I took my shoes off in a cloakroom, then ventured into a large kitchen where little Indian statues of couples in coitus sat beside generic holiday snaps of Cliff's children.

Trays and bowls of food were arrayed on countertops – a buffet of the type you would find in the business lounge of a regional airport: grapes and apple slices and small slabs of cheese – but there was cling film over them. It wasn't yet time to eat.

The kitchen filled up: couples, a handful of singles, male and female in roughly equal measure, most in their thirties and forties.

Many of the guys were in plain collared shirts, and the women in knee-length dresses – they might have been at a church mixer.

But there was also a sprinkling of more flamboyant partygoers. A bearded man in a blue sarong, his shirt unbuttoned to show a huge blue pendant resplendent on his hairy chest. Another, older, dreadlocked man, in black leggings and a little leatherette waistcoat. A heavyset lady in an orange kimono that was open to reveal a generous helping of cleavage.

A woman, probably in her thirties, was smiling at me with a daffy air of free-spirited bonhomie that seemed to invite further inquiry.

'Are you excited?' I asked.

'I'm *so* excited!' she replied.

'Are you nervous too?'

'Nuh! Why would someone be nervous? It's just a night of fun and freedom! It's all about the pleasure.'

'Yeah, the pleasure – of the food,' I added hopefully.

'Yeah! Well, you know, the food *and* . . .' Eyes wide, she trailed off.

'Have you been fed food before?' asked a grey-haired older lady with dangly earrings. She placed her hand on my chest. 'I think you're going to really enjoy the experience. You're pretty safe. We're a good group of people.'

'Oh, it's good to hear that,' I said.

At Cliff's direction, we separated into three groups. Group one began loading up plates with food and pouring drinks into plastic beakers with sippy-cup lids. Then we all made our way downstairs to a basement where mats were laid out and gentle music was playing.

'As those who have been to my events before – the massage-à-trois, the tantra events – know, I'm really into putting together events where you learn something about yourself,' Cliff said. 'You learn to connect more deeply. This is an L2 event, so genitals stay covered. No genital touching. But whatever else you would like to take off, feel free to take off. If you don't have any underwear I've got plenty of my sarongs you can wear.'

Group one sat down with their plates and beakers next to them. Some took their tops off.

'If you like what's happening, say yes. If you really like it, say yes please,' Cliff said. 'If you're feeling overwhelmed and you need a pause say "ground".'

Then, at Cliff's command, group one put eye masks on, and Cliff said it was time to start.

It was a little like a starter's pistol had gone off but, instead of running in a straight direction, the masked athletes began swaying and groaning with their mouths open like little baby chicks, as the non-masked party-goers – the 'feeders' – set about massaging and stroking and, well, feeding.

'Givers, feed slowly,' Cliff said. 'Feed off part of your body but do everything slowly. Slow is always better.'

I was immediately feeling a little out of my depth. *Oh Christ*, I thought. I did my best to go with the flow, circulating slightly aimlessly, trying to stay in the orbit of receivers who already had a giver next to them, to take the pressure off me. But even with a two-to-one ratio, it still occasionally happened that I was left alone with a receiver, which induced mild feelings of panic, having the sole responsibility of imparting profound feelings of connectedness and emotional well-being. In a way the feeding was the easy part: you pop a chocolate in someone's mouth, they go 'mmm!' But you can't just keep feeding and feeding, and it wasn't totally clear what the next move was: you squeeze the shoulders, massage the arms a little bit, but then what? I was running out of ideas. A bit more chocolate? A strawberry?

As the minutes passed, there was a palpable escalation in the groaning and gyrating. Cliff was keeping up a patter of encouragement. 'Find connection on a deeper level,' he intoned as he paced up and down. Across from me, a long-haired woman, who I knew to be a doctor, was squirting whipped cream onto one of her breasts and with a big smile on her face feeding it – the cream and possibly portions of breast – to her receiver. Meanwhile the man in the leatherette waistcoat was moaning and spasming in ecstasy. I looked over at my director Arron to try to gauge his reaction: was this what he'd been expecting? His eye was fixed to his camera.

And then it was my turn: group two was called. And what, after all, was I doing here if I wasn't going to get involved? I loaded my plate with some chocolate, some strawberries, slices of apple. I'd heard someone recommend a combination of savoury and sweet, so I added a couple of slabs of cheese. I took my shirt off, and I put my eye mask on, noticing a strange sense of liberation as my vision was obscured. I felt invisible and some of my self-consciousness ebbed away.

'Human connection is one of the most precious things we can experience in our lives,' Cliff was saying. 'This is an incredibly safe space to explore touch, to explore sensuality.'

Strawberries and cream were tickling around my mouth. I was aware of a low throaty sound and a soft face pressing against my cheeks. Then a warm hairy body was at my back – I had the impression of a pendant and then more flavours: chocolate, whipped cream. I was saying my 'yeses' and 'thank yous'; there was the sensation of other bodies and bits of chocolate and more strawberries entering my mouth and cheese – possibly a little too much cheese, though I didn't like to mention it because I thought it might spoil the mood – and above all there was a growing feeling of connectedness, the faint echo of the tingling sensation of a first kiss with a new lover. I had to admit I was enjoying it.

And then it was all over. I took my mask off to see Cliff sambaing up and down in a transport of satisfaction at the tableau he had created. But for a moment the idea of a community in which the currency of sex and love was more free-flowing made a tiny bit of sense. I rubbed my eyes at a world that felt a little friendlier, a little closer to home.

A little later I said my goodbyes and drove back to my hotel with the crew. In the minivan I felt slightly sheepish at how far I'd gone with my commitment to experiencing the workshop. I had the familiar sensation of being assailed by multiple ironies, of having been in control of an experience and at the same time out of my depth. I thought about my wife, Nancy, aware that the scene I'd told her we'd be filming – involving me being fed a couple of strawberries by scantily clad women – had turned out to be more outré than I'd expected. I wondered whether she would be upset and annoyed.

And I thought, here I am, aged forty-seven, still making a fool of myself for the purposes of a TV show, creating connections in unlikely places, in a spirit in which the boundaries between silliness and seriousness, sincerity and role-playing, self-exposure and canny journalistic revelation weren't always clear even to me. Here I am, telling stories, using myself, my feelings, for real – after so many years, still doing it.